Atlas of Coronary Intravascular Optical Coherence Tomography

Annapoorna Kini • Jagat Narula
Yuliya Vengrenyuk • Samin Sharma

Atlas of Coronary Intravascular Optical Coherence Tomography

Springer

Annapoorna Kini
Director, Cardiac Catheterization Laboratory
Director, Structural Heart Intervention Program
Director, Interventional Cardiology Fellowship Program
Zena and Michael A. Wiener Professor of Medicine
Icahn School of Medicine at Mount Sinai
Mount Sinai Hospital
New York, NY
USA

Yuliya Vengrenyuk
Director, Intravascular Imaging Core Laboratory
Instructor, Department of Medicine
Icahn School of Medicine at Mount Sinai
Mount Sinai Hospital
New York, NY
USA

Jagat Narula
Philip J. and Harriet L. Goodhart Chair in Cardiology
Chief of Cardiology, Mount Sinai St. Luke's Hospital
Professor of Medicine and Radiology
Associate Dean, Arnhold Institute for Global Health
Icahn School of Medicine at Mount Sinai
Mount Sinai Hospital
New York, NY
USA

Samin Sharma
Director, Clinical and Interventional Cardiology
President, Mount Sinai Heart Network
Dean, International Clinical Affiliations
Anandi Lal Sharma Professor of Medicine
Icahn School of Medicine at Mount Sinai
Mount Sinai Hospital
New York, NY
USA

ISBN 978-3-319-62664-2 ISBN 978-3-319-62666-6 (eBook)
DOI 10.1007/978-3-319-62666-6

Library of Congress Control Number: 2017951871

Printed on acid-free paper

This Springer imprint is published by Springer Nature
The registered company is Springer International Publishing AG
The registered company address is: Gewerbestrasse 11, 6330 Cham, Switzerland

Preface

Optical coherence tomography (OCT) is an emerging intravascular imaging modality, which allows to visualize the coronary pathophysiology in vivo with unprecedented detail and clarity almost comparable to histology. While many hundreds of studies have been published utilizing coronary artery OCT, very few have focused on its application in day-to-day clinical practice. The cardiac catheterization laboratory at the Mount Sinai Hospital in New York is proud to share best practices for improving outcomes in complex coronary cases. We conduct teaching classes every day, use webcasts for live cases watched across the world by more than 6000 cardiologists once every month, and hold two large symposia every year to help drive best practices among interventional cardiologists and fellows of the catheterization laboratory. OCT is being evaluated as a promising intravascular imaging modality that may contribute immensely to niche areas in percutaneous coronary intervention (PCI) and clinical trials.

This Atlas is a practical and illustrated guide to the use of intravascular OCT in diagnosis and management of coronary artery disease. The first introduction chapter provides a systematic introduction to intracoronary imaging with OCT. It also explains how to interpret images and describes abnormal findings seen in atherosclerosis and stent assessment. The following chapters present real-life case studies that show how OCT could be used in clinical practice in an academic center to better address a diagnostic dilemma and complications of interventional procedure, select appropriate treatment, and evaluate complications and results. Each case includes a brief clinical history, procedural summary, angiography with OCT images, and a discussion of how OCT influenced the clinical decision-making process. OCT imaging pullbacks before and after intervention are available online for the majority of cases. In addition to OCT, intravascular ultrasound (IVUS) and near-infrared spectroscopy (NIRS) images of the same lesions are available for a subset of cases.

New York, NY, USA	Annapoorna Kini
New York, NY, USA	Jagat Narula
New York, NY, USA	Yuliya Vengrenyuk
New York, NY, USA	Samin Sharma

Contents

Abbreviations

ACS	Acute coronary syndrome
BMS	Bare metal stent
BRS	Bioresorbable vascular scaffold
CABG	Coronary artery bypass grafting
CaN	Calcified nodule
CB	Cutting balloon
CCS	Canadian Cardiovascular Society
CSA	Cross sectional area
CTA	Computed tomography angiography
cTnI	Cardiac troponin I
CTO	Chronic total occlusion
D1	First diagonal branch
DES	Drug-eluting stent
DM	Diabetes mellitus
ECG	Electrocardiography
EEM	External elastic membrane
FFR	Fractional flow reserve
FL	False lumen
IDDM	Insulin-dependent diabetes mellitus
ISR	In-stent restenosis
IVUS	Intravascular ultrasound
KBI	Kissing balloon inflation
LAD	Left anterior descending artery
LCBI	Lipid core burden index
LCX	Left circumflex artery
LIMA	Left internal mammary artery
LM	Left main artery
MACE	Major adverse cardiac events
MI	Myocardial infarction
MLA	Minimal lumen area
MSA	Minimal stent area
NIDDM	Non-insulin-dependent diabetes mellitus
NIRS	Near infrared spectroscopy
NSTEMI	Non-ST-elevation myocardial infarction
OA	Orbital atherectomy
OCT	Optical coherence tomography
OFDI	Optical frequency domain imaging
PCI	Percutaneous coronary intervention
PER	Plaque erosion
PRU	Plaque rupture
RA	Rotational atherectomy
RCA	Right coronary artery

RI	Ramus intermedius
Rpm	Revolutions Per Minute
SBOA	Side branch ostium area
SCAD	Spontaneous coronary artery dissection
SCD	Sudden cardiac death
SLE	Systemic lupus erythematous
SPECT MPI	Single-photon emission computed tomography myocardial perfusion imaging
ST	Stent thrombosis
STEMI	ST-elevation myocardial infarction
TIMI	Thrombolysis in myocardial infarction

List of Videos

1 Optical Coherence Tomography: Principles, Image Acquisition, and Assessment

1.1 Optical Coherence Tomography Principles

Optical coherence tomography (OCT) uses near-infrared light to generate high-resolution images of coronary arteries in vivo [1, 2] and can be considered an optical analog of intravascular ultrasound, which uses light instead of sound. The near-infrared light with a wavelength of about 1.3 μm is invisible to the human eye. OCT uses low-coherence interferometry by measuring the echo time delay and intensity of the light reflected from internal structures in tissue to generate cross-sectional images. The light beam from an OCT system is split by an interferometer into two arms, a sample arm and a reference arm. The sample arm light travels to the sample tissue, then is being reflected, refracted, or absorbed by the tissue and finally travels back to the interferometer. The reference arm is directed to a mirror, which reflects it back to the interferometer, combined with the sample arm light and detected by a detector. The OCT image is built based on the interaction between these two light waves, depending on whether there is constructive or destructive interference between the waves [1]. Cross-sectional images are generated by measuring the delay time and intensity of light reflected or backscattered from internal structures in biologic tissue [1, 3, 4]. There are two types of OCT systems: first generation time domain (TD-OCT) and second generation frequency domain (FD-OCT) (Fig. 1.1) [5, 6]. A reference arm and an interferometer are used by both systems to detect echo time delays of light. While the reference arm in TD-OCT is mechanically scanned by a moving mirror to produce a time-varying time delay, the light source is frequency swept in FD-OCT. As a result, the interference of the light beam from tissue and reference oscillates according to the frequency difference. The main limitation of first TD-OCT systems was the need for an occlusion balloon inflated proximally to the imaged segment to remove blood from the vessel. Since FD-OCT systems use fixed reference mirror and adjustable laser light sources with a wavelength between 1250 and 1370 nm, they can reach a much higher imaging speed, eliminating the need for an occlusive balloon. A summary of physical characteristics of FD-OCT and TD-OCT compared to intravascular ultrasound (IVUS) is shown in Table 1.1. While OCT can produce images with a resolution of 10–20 μm, an order of magnitude higher compared to IVUS, it cannot image through blood, since blood attenuates near-infrared light and therefore clearing of blood from the lumen is required. In addition, the penetration depth of OCT usually ranges between 1 and 3 mm depending on tissue type, which prevents visualizing external elastic membrane in large lesions [7].

A. Kini et al., *Atlas of Coronary Intravascular Optical Coherence Tomography*, DOI 10.1007/978-3-319-62666-6_1

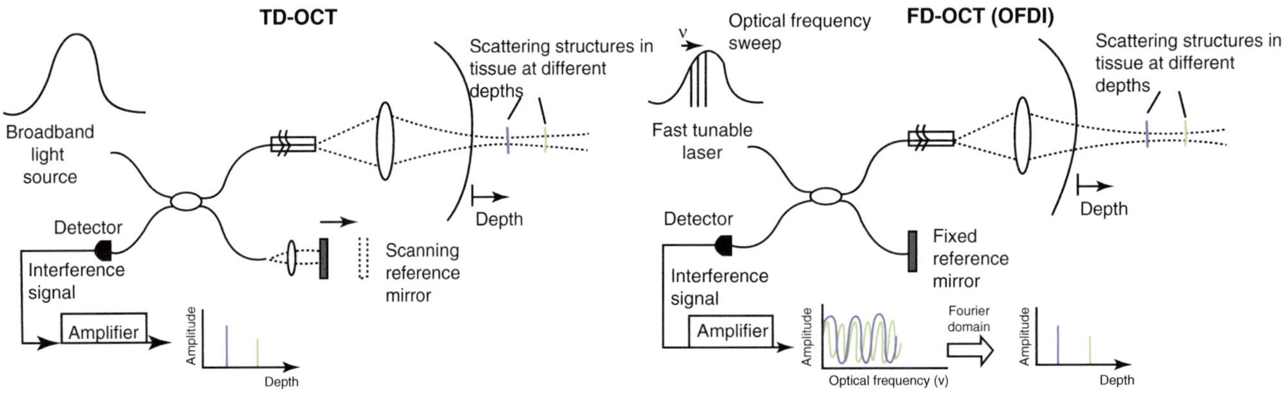

Fig. 1.1 Schematic representation of time-domain optical coherence tomography (TD-OCT, *left panel*) and frequency or Fourier-domain optical coherence tomography (FD-OCT, *right panel*). (*Adapted from* Bezerra et al. [5])

Table 1.1 Comparison of IVUS and OCT

	IVUS	TD OCT	FD OCT
Energy wave	Ultrasound	Near-infrared	Near-infrared
Wavelength, μm	35–80	1.3	1.3
Resolution, axial/lateral, μm	100/200	15/90	15/20–40
Frame rate, frames/s	30	16–20	100
Pullback rate, mm/s	0.5–1.0	1–3	20
Axial scans × 1000	–	3.2–4.8	5.4
Lines, axial scans/frame	–	200–40	500
Maximum scan diameter, mm	10	6.8	9.7
Tissue penetration, mm	10	1–2.5	2.0–3.5

Reprinted from Lowe et al. [7]; *with permission*

1.2 Equipment

An OCT catheter contains a rotating single-mode optical fiber with a lens and refractor element at its distal end to focus the beam and direct it sideways into the vessel wall [6]. The catheter is connected to a rotary junction with a motor unit to rotate the fiber. Currently available imaging probes for TD-OCT have a maximal outer diameter of 0.019 in. and contain a single-mode fiberoptic core within a translucent sheath. The imaging probes for FD-OCT are integrated in a short monorail catheter comparable to conventional 0.014 in. angioplasty guidewires and 6 Fr or larger guiding catheters. The reflected light signal is detected and converted to digital signals within an OCT console. The console can also be used to control the rotational and pullback speed of the catheter. Finally, it allows adjustment of Z-offset, a variation in the optical path length of the optical fiber within the catheter, by performing calibration before each OCT imaging in order to avoid errors in OCT measurements.

1.3 Image Acquisition and Safety

Similar to the IVUS procedure, patients undergoing OCT imaging require systemic anticoagulation with heparin before the guidewire is inserted into the vessel [6]. In order to avoid catheter-induced vasospasm, image acquisition is performed after administration of intracoronary nitroglycerin. OCT imaging is performed with caution in patients with severely impaired left ventricular function, markedly impaired renal function, a single remaining vessel, or known allergy to contrast media. OCT imaging can be conducted using either manual or motorized pullback. Proper blood clearing during image acquisition is crucial for obtaining good quality images, since infra-red light cannot penetrate blood. There are two blood clearing techniques for TD-OCT, the occlusive and nonocclusive approaches. While the majority of occlusive TD-OCT procedures have been performed using the occlusive method requiring balloon inflation proximal to the lesion, the nonocclusive technique has become a more popular acquisition method with recent improvements in the acquisition speed of TD-OCT. FD-OCT is mostly performed with the nonocclusive flushing technique, which allows reduction of potential myocardial ischemia and vessel injury due to balloon inflation. First, a standard intracoronary guidewire (0.014″) is used to cross the target lesion; then, the OCT probe is positioned over the guidewire distal to the lesion. A pullback is performed manually or automatically (10–40 mm/s) with simultaneous injection of a bolus of contrast agent through the guiding catheter. The infusion rate is usually set to 2–4 mL/s, depending on the artery. Automated contrast injection might help optimize image quality, since the pullback would start automatically only if blood clearance is recognized distally. A proper guiding catheter engagement, coaxially and deeply in the ostium, is important for obtaining high quality images. A manual injection of a small bolus of contrast agent before imaging can be used in order to verify good guide catheter position. Several recent technical developments have dramatically reduced imaging times, resulting in a very short injection sufficient for optimal image acquisition.

In a multicenter registry of 468 consecutive patients who underwent TD-OCT imaging, major complications included five cases of ventricular fibrillation caused by balloon occlusion and/or deep guide catheter intubation, three cases of air embolism, and one case of vessel dissection [8]. There were no cases of coronary spasm or major adverse cardiovascular event during or within the 24-h period following OCT imaging. There were no major complications reported with FD-OCT using nonocclusive flushing in a small feasibility study [9] and a larger single center registry [10], suggesting that FD-OCT is a feasible and safe technique for guidance of coronary interventions. Both occlusive and nonocclusive OCT image acquisition were demonstrated to be safe in several studies [11, 12].

1.4 Image Display and Assessment

The normal vessel wall is characterized by a layered architecture (Fig. 1.2). In the presence of atherosclerotic plaque, the lumen usually appears narrowed, and the layered structure of the vessel wall is deranged (Fig. 1.3). Plaques can be characterized as fibrous, lipid-rich, or calcified, according to plaque characterization criteria developed by histology validation studies [6, 13, 14]. Fibrous plaque appears on OCT imaging as a relatively homogeneous signal-rich region (Fig. 1.3a, b). Calcification is characterized by a signal-poor area with sharply delineated borders (Fig. 1.3c, d). In contrast, lipid-rich plaque appears as a signal-poor region with diffuse borders and an overlying signal-rich layer and a fibrous cap (Fig. 1.4). The low intensity areas with poorly defined outlines correspond to the necrotic core. OCT thin-capped fibroatheroma is a lipid-rich plaque with the minimal fibrous cap thickness less than a predetermined threshold. The most commonly used cutoff of 65 μm is defined by pathology studies [15]. Vessels within the intima may be visualized by OCT as sharply delineated signal-poor voids (Fig. 1.5a). Macrophage accumulation can appear as signal-rich either distinct or confluent punctate regions significantly attenuating the OCT signal (Fig. 1.5b). Cholesterol crystals appear as thin linear signal-rich structures with low signal attenuation (Fig. 1.5c, d). Plaque rupture is defined as a lipid-rich plaque with fibrous cap discontinuity and formation of a cavity inside the plaque (Fig. 1.6a). In contrast, OCT plaque erosion does not show any evidence of cap disruption (Fig. 1.6b). A thrombus is identified by OCT as a protruding mass attached to a luminal surface or floating within the lumen (Fig. 1.7). OCT can differentiate between red cell–rich red and platelet-rich white thrombi. Stent malapposition, underexpansion, dissections, tissue prolapse, and thrombi are the most common immediate findings after stent implantation (Fig. 1.8). OCT can provide unique micron-scale level insights into stent strut coverage for follow-up imaging and characterize the morphology of an in-stent restenosis lesion (Fig. 1.9). An important part of image interpretation is understanding and recognizing OCT imaging artifacts (Fig. 1.10) [5, 6].

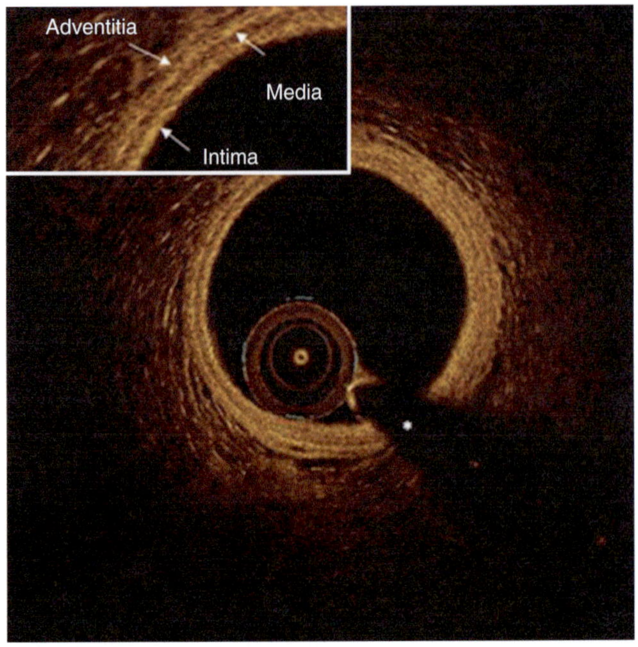

Fig. 1.2 OCT findings in healthy coronary arteries. In normal vessels, the coronary artery wall demonstrates a three-layered structure consisting of a signal poor muscular media layer between high backscattering thin intima and a heterogeneous and frequently highly backscattering adventitia as shown in the magnified image box. The dark band of media is delimited by the internal elastic membrane (IEM) and external elastic membrane (EEM), two thin layers of elastic fibers at the border between the intima and media, the media and adventitia. The highly backscattering thin layers sometimes can be visualized by OCT. *Guidewire artifact

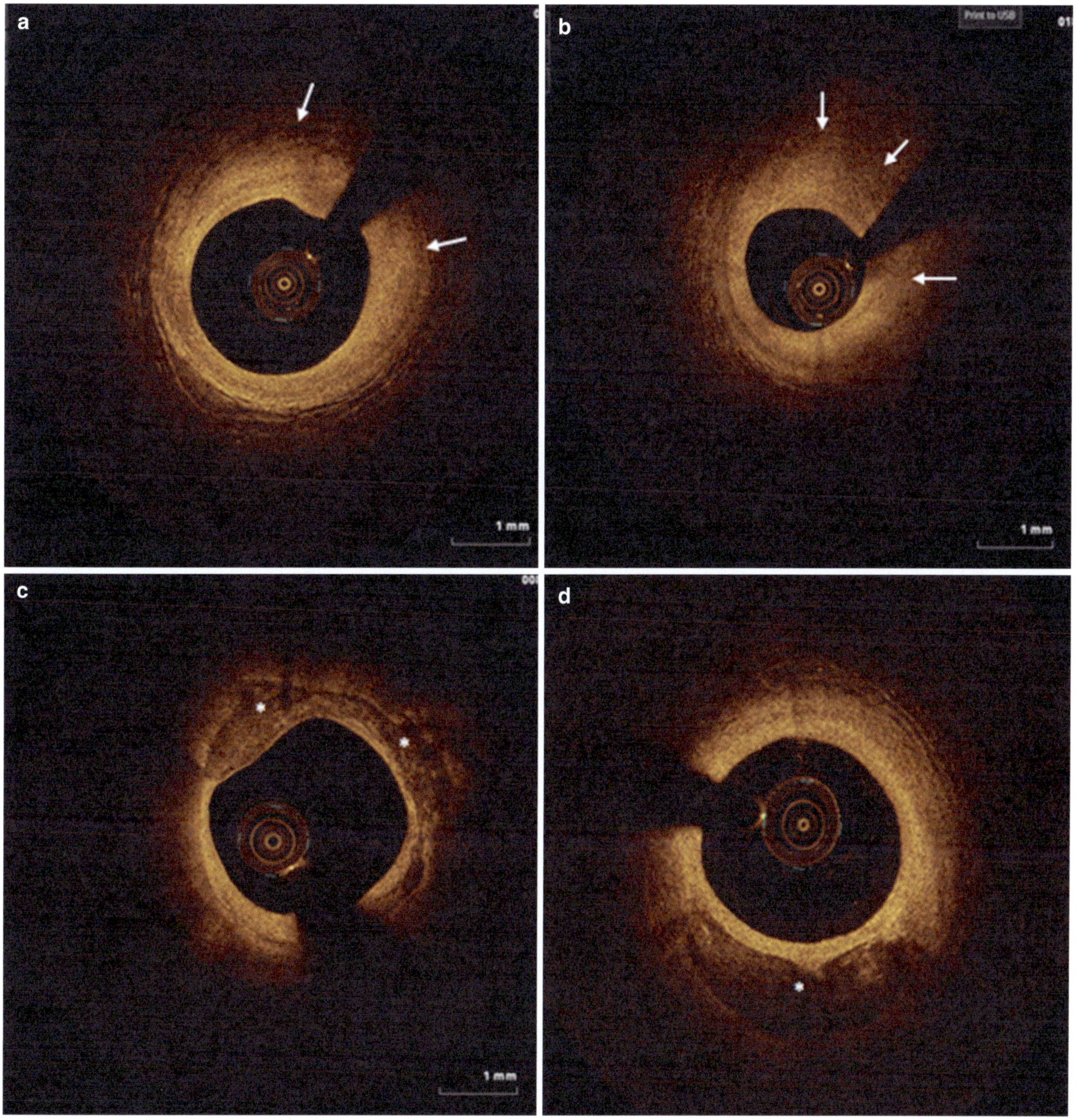

Fig. 1.3 A fibrous coronary plaque is characterized by a high backscattering and a relatively homogeneous signal (**a** and **b**, *arrows*). In some fibrous plaques, IEM and EEM can be visualized by OCT (**a**). If either of the two elastic layers cannot be identified in a lesion (**b**), there might be deep lipid or calcification behind the thick layer of fibrous tissue, the accurate detection of which is not possible because of the limited penetration depth of OCT. In addition to fibrous tissue, fibrocalcific plaque demonstrates the presence of calcification that appears as a signal-poor region with sharply delineated borders (**c** and **d**, *asterisks*)

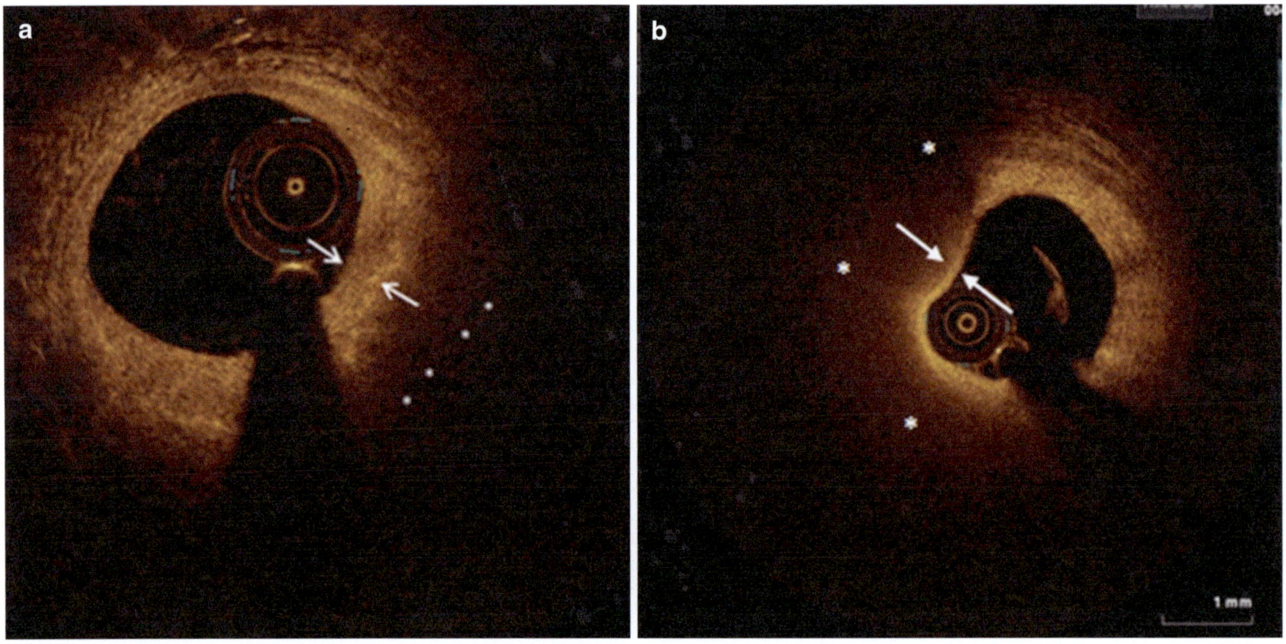

Fig. 1.4 Thick and thin-cap fibroatheromas. A necrotic core by OCT is a poorly delineated region with fast signal drop-off and very little OCT signal backscattering (*asterisks*). The fibrous cap is a signal-rich tissue layer overlying a signal-poor necrotic core (**a** and **b**, *arrows*). The fibroatheroma is a coronary lesion with a fibrous cap and a necrotic core. The OCT thin-capped fibroatheroma (TCFA) is a fibroatheroma with a minimal cap thickness less than a predetermined threshold, usually 65 μm (**b**, *arrows*)

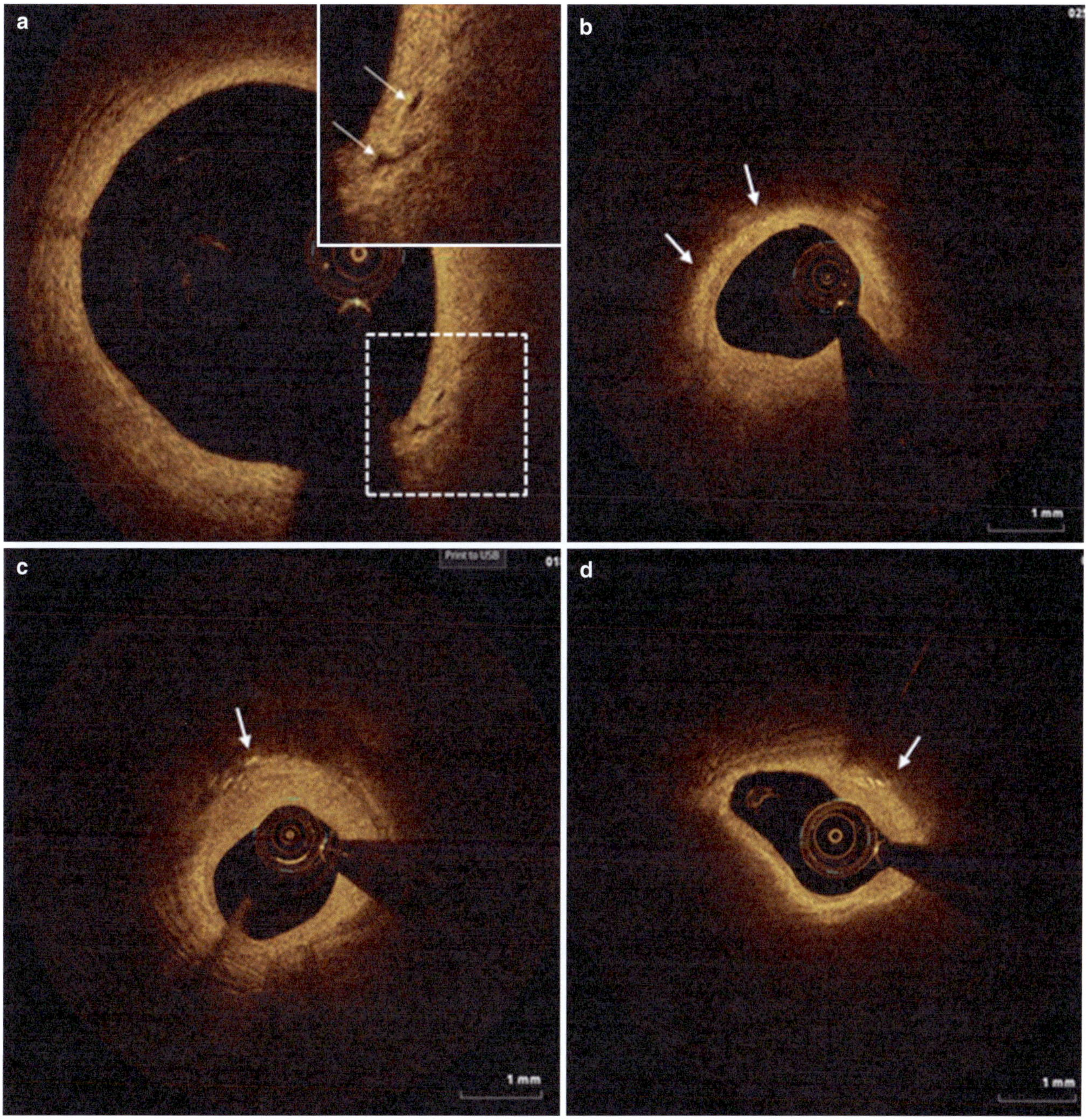

Fig. 1.5 Intimal vasculature, macrophage accumulation, and cholesterol crystals. Vessels in the intima may be seen by OCT as sharply delineated signal-poor voids, which can be traced in multiple continuous frames (**a**). Macrophages appear as signal-rich punctate focal regions that exceed the background intensity (**b**). They are often found at the boundary between the fibrous cap and the necrotic core. Superficial macrophages can shadow underlying tissue, creating an appearance of a necrotic core. Cholesterol crystals appear as linear regions of high intensity, most often associated with a fibrous cap and necrotic core (**c** and **d**)

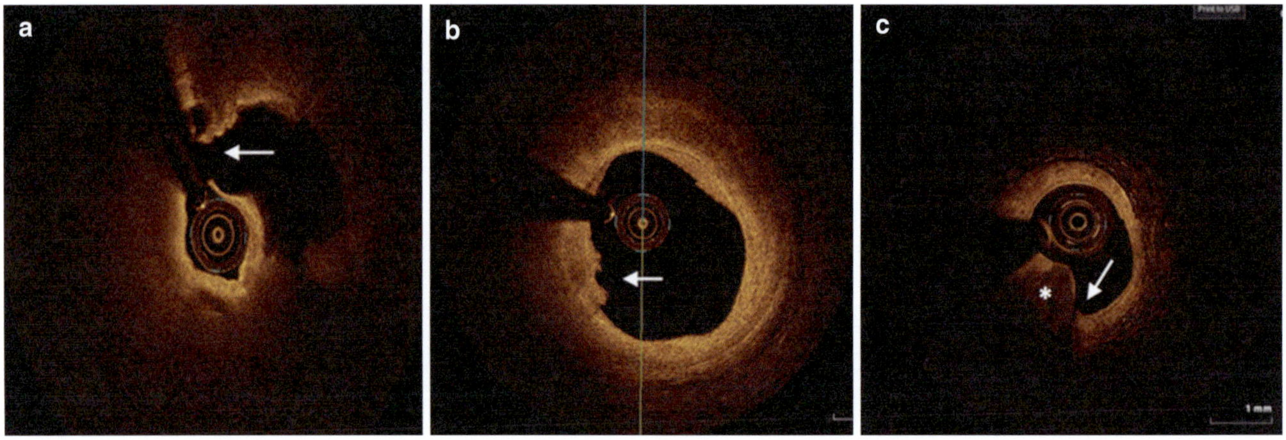

Fig. 1.6 Plaque rupture, plaque erosion, and calcific nodule. Ruptured plaques show features of intimal tearing or fibrous cap disruption and are frequently observed in TCFA lesions with or without a superimposed thrombus (**a**, *arrow*). Plaque erosion is characterized by the presence of a thrombus on an irregular luminal surface and no evidence of fibrous cap rupture (**b**). A calcified nodule demonstrates fibrous cap disruption (*arrow*) and single or multiple regions of calcium protruding into the lumen (**c**, *asterisk*)

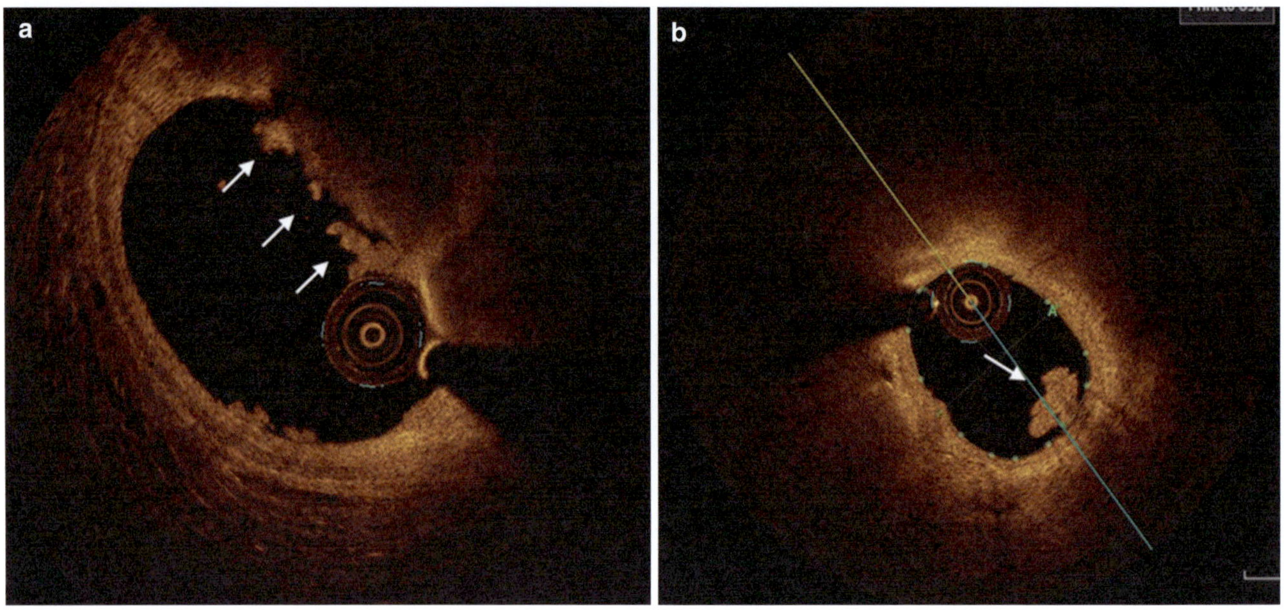

Fig. 1.7 OCT examples of red and white thrombi. The thrombus by OCT can appear as a mass either attached to the vessel lumen or floating within it (**a** and **b**). The OCT is capable of discriminating two different types of thrombi: red, red blood–cell rich (**a**) and white, platelet-rich thrombus (**b**). The red thrombus appears as a highly backscattering intravascular mass, which has high signal attenuation resulting in shadowing, since red blood cells attenuate OCT signal (**a**). The shadowing can obscure underlying vascular structure. The white thrombus is less backscattering and produces little signal attenuation; underlying vessel structure can be easily visualized (**b**)

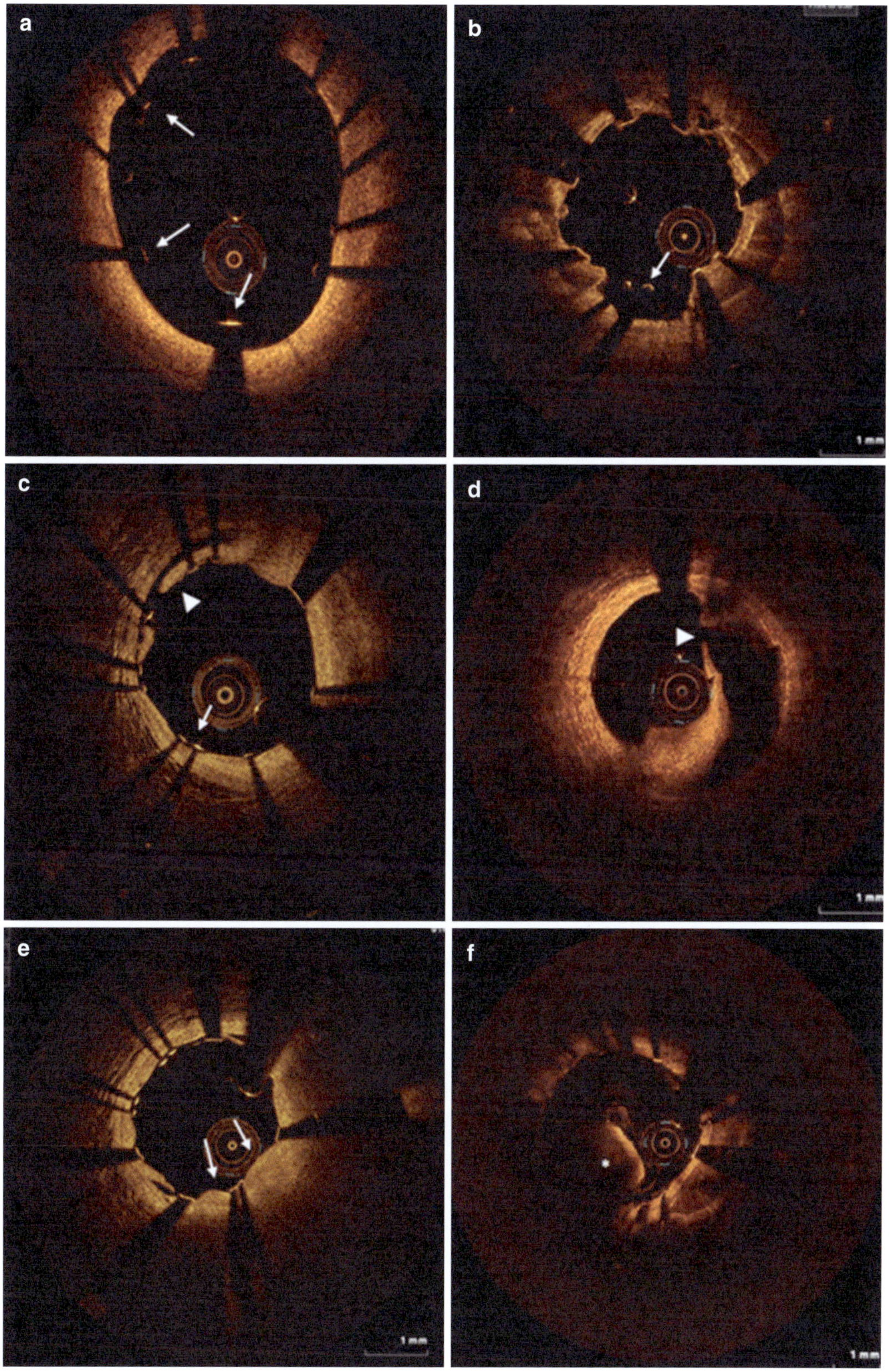

Fig. 1.8 OCT findings after coronary stenting. Metallic stent struts appear as bright structures with dorsal shadowing (**a–c**, *arrows*). Stent malapposition is present when the distance between the strut and the luminal surface is greater than the strut thickness (**a**, *arrows*). Intra-stent dissection is characterized by a disruption of the lumen surface inside the stent (**c**, *arrowhead*). Stent edge dissection appears as a disruption of the lumen surface at the edge of the stent without visible struts (**d**, *arrowhead*). Tissue prolapse is represented by a convex-shaped protrusion of tissue between the stent struts without disruption of the intima (**e**, *arrows*). In-stent thrombus is defined as a mass protruding into the lumen through the stent struts usually characterized by significant attenuation (**f**, *asterisk*)

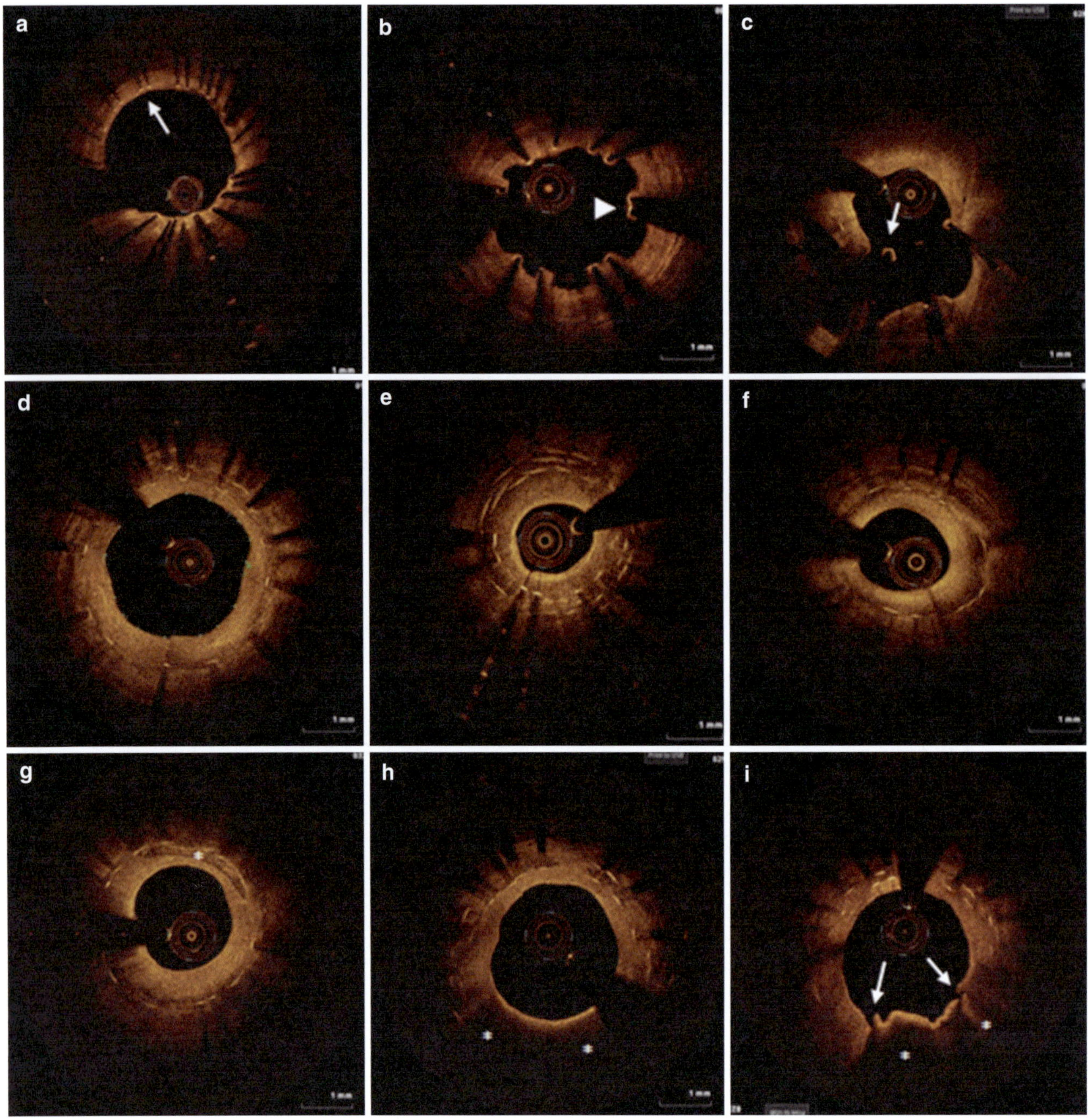

Fig. 1.9 Stent strut coverage and in-stent restenosis. Struts can be classified into covered (**a**, *arrow*) and uncovered (**b**, *arrowhead*), based on the presence of the overlying tissue. Some of the struts "hanging" over a side branch appear covered (**c**, *arrow*). For stent restenosis, OCT can characterize different patterns of neointimal tissue as homogeneous (**d**), heterogeneous (**e**), and layered (**f**), with the majority of the lesions characterized by high backscatter and appearing bright [16]. In some cases, when the neointima demonstrates the presence of atherosclerosis, OCT can differentiate between calcified (**g**, *asterisk*) and lipid-laden neointima (**h** and **i**, *asterisks*) with neointimal disruption (**i**, *arrows*)

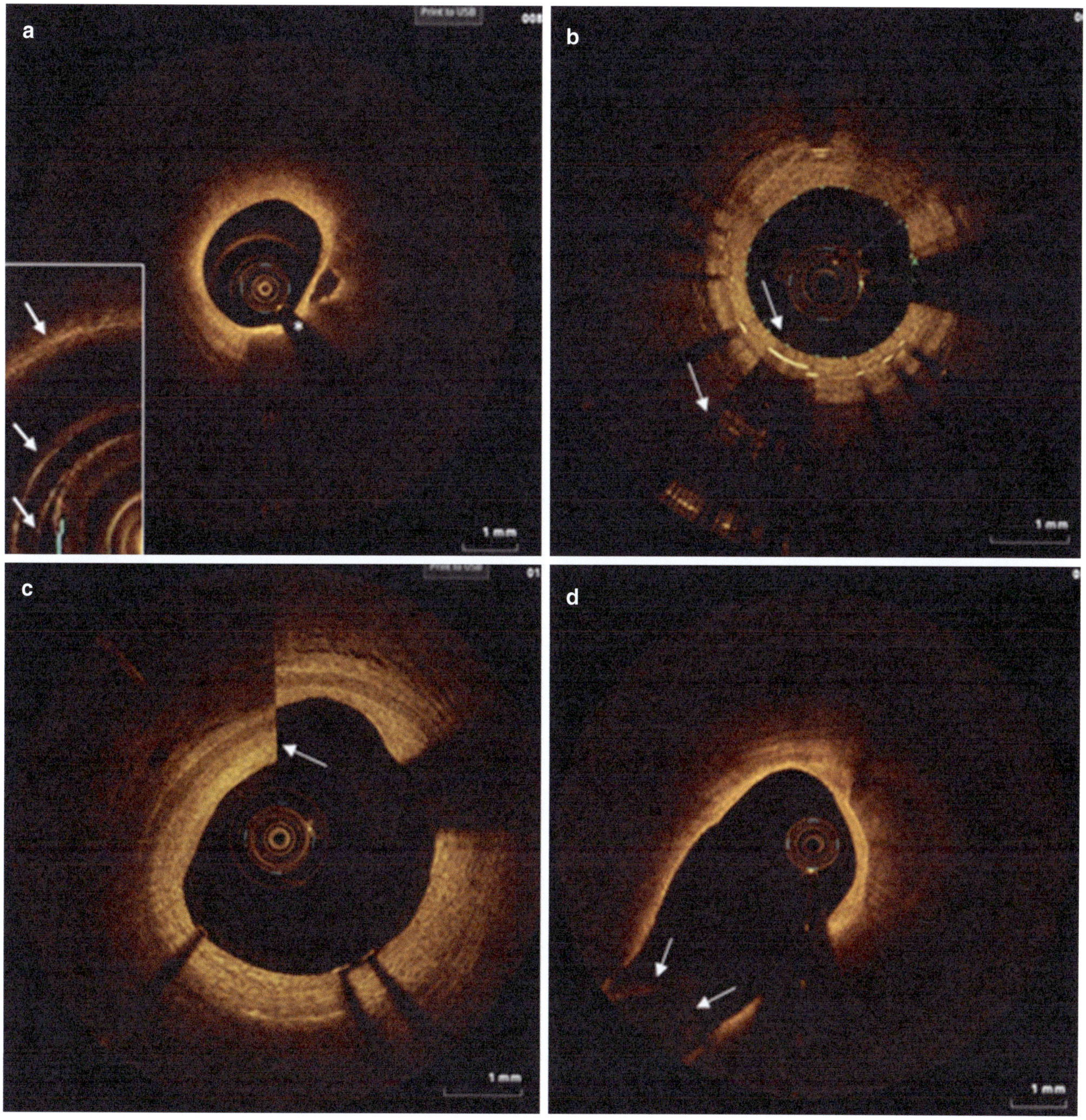

Fig. 1.10 OCT imaging artifacts. *Guidewire artifact*. A shadow from the guidewire visualized in all OCT images completely masks the underlying plaque or stent features (**a**, *asterisk*). *Multiple reflections*. One or more circular lines can appear as a result of light reflecting from the catheter surfaces (**a**, *arrows*). Using these lines for calibration instead of the catheter edge can lead to incorrect measurements. *Saturation artifact* can be observed as bright lines along the axial direction when the intensity of the backscattered signal is too high to be accurately detected by the OCT detector (**b**, *arrows*). Metallic stent struts and the guidewire are the most common structures exhibiting high backscattering. *Sew-up artifact* may appear as a result of the catheter movement during a single cross-section acquisition time characterized by formation of a seam line (**c**, *arrow*). *Fold-over artifact* can be observed in large vessels and around side branches and appears as a portion of the vessel folded over in the image (**d**, *arrows*). *Residual blood* in the vessel attenuates the OCT signal and may result in unacceptable image quality (**e**) compared to the second pullback of the same lesion with optimal vessel flushing (**f**). In some cases, the image quality is sufficient to visualize some features, but objects imaged through blood may appear dimmer and larger (**g**, *arrow*) than expected (**h**, *arrow*), leading *to scattering* and *focus artifacts*. Care should be taken while interpreting images with suboptimal blood clearance, since blood within the lumen can be misinterpreted as a thrombus. *Tangential signal dropout*. When the OCT catheter is located close to the vessel wall, the light beam is directed almost parallel to the lumen surface, resulting in signal attenuation while passing along the surface of the vessel wall. A signal-poor area within the artery wall may appear as a result of the catheter position (**i**, *asterisk*). In order to avoid image misinterpretation, tangential signal dropout artifact should be taken into account whenever the imaging beam strikes the vessel under a glancing angle owing to the catheter position. A dark radial feature can be also observed at the site of glancing incidence (**j**, *arrow*) [17]

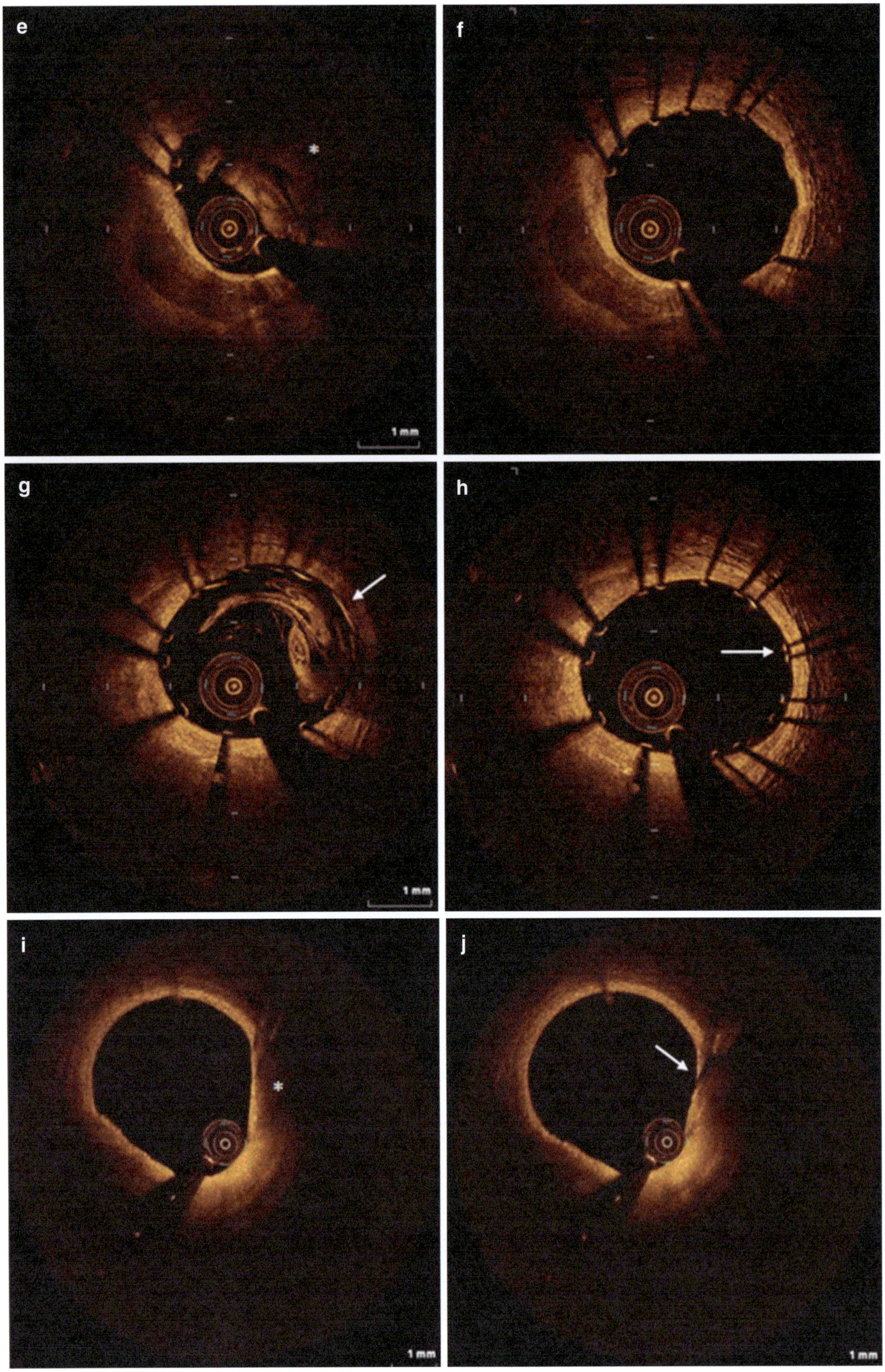

Fig. 1.10 (continued)

References

1. Huang D, Swanson EA, Lin CP, Schuman JS, Stinson WG, Chang W, et al. Optical coherence tomography. Science. 1991;254:1178–81.
2. Brezinski ME, Tearney GJ, Bouma BE, Izatt JA, Hee MR, Swanson EA, et al. Optical coherence tomography for optical biopsy. Properties and demonstration of vascular pathology. Circulation. 1996;93:1206–13.
3. Tearney GJ, Brezinski ME, Bouma BE, Boppart SA, Pitris C, Southern JF, Fujimoto JG. In vivo endoscopic optical biopsy with optical coherence tomography. Science. 1997;276:2037–9.
4. Jang IK, Bouma BE, Kang DH, Park SJ, Park SW, Seung KB, et al. Visualization of coronary atherosclerotic plaques in patients using optical coherence tomography: comparison with intravascular ultrasound. J Am Coll Cardiol. 2002;39:604–9.
5. Bezerra HG, Costa MA, Guagliumi G, Rollins AM, Simon DI. Intracoronary optical coherence tomography: a comprehensive review clinical and research applications. JACC Cardiovasc Interv. 2009;2:1035–46.
6. Tearney GJ, Regar E, Akasaka T, Adriaenssens T, Barlis P, Bezerra HG, et al. Consensus standards for acquisition, measurement, and reporting of intravascular optical coherence tomography studies: a report from the International Working Group for Intravascular Optical Coherence Tomography Standardization and Validation. J Am Coll Cardiol. 2012;59:1058–72.
7. Lowe HC, Narula J, Fujimoto JG, Jang IK. Intracoronary optical diagnostics current status, limitations, and potential. JACC Cardiovasc Interv. 2011;4:1257–70.
8. Barlis P, Gonzalo N, Di Mario C, Prati F, Buellesfeld L, Rieber J, et al. A multicentre evaluation of the safety of intracoronary optical coherence tomography. EuroIntervention. 2009;5:90–5.
9. Takarada S, Imanishi T, Liu Y, Ikejima H, Tsujioka H, Kuroi A, et al. Advantage of next-generation frequency-domain optical coherence tomography compared with conventional time-domain system in the assessment of coronary lesion. Catheter Cardiovasc Interv. 2010;75:202–6.
10. Imola F, Mallus MT, Ramazzotti V, Manzoli A, Pappalardo A, Di Giorgio A, et al. Safety and feasibility of frequency domain optical coherence tomography to guide decision making in percutaneous coronary intervention. EuroIntervention. 2010;6:575–81.
11. Prati F, Cera M, Ramazzotti V, Imola F, Giudice R, Albertucci M. Safety and feasibility of a new non-occlusive technique for facilitated intracoronary optical coherence tomography (OCT) acquisition in various clinical and anatomical scenarios. EuroIntervention. 2007;3:365–70.
12. Yamaguchi T, Terashima M, Akasaka T, Hayashi T, Mizuno K, Muramatsu T, et al. Safety and feasibility of an intravascular optical coherence tomography image wire system in the clinical setting. Am J Cardiol. 2008;101:562–7.
13. Yabushita H, Bouma BE, Houser SL, Aretz HT, Jang IK, Schlendorf KH, et al. Characterization of human atherosclerosis by optical coherence tomography. Circulation. 2002;106:1640–5.
14. Kume T, Akasaka T, Kawamoto T, Watanabe N, Toyota E, Neishi Y, et al. Assessment of coronary arterial plaque by optical coherence tomography. Am J Cardiol. 2006;97:1172–5.
15. Virmani R, Burke AP, Farb A, Kolodgie FD. Pathology of the vulnerable plaque. J Am Coll Cardiol. 2006;47:C13–8.
16. Gonzalo N, Serruys PW, Okamura T, van Beusekom HM, Garcia-Garcia HM, van Soest G, et al. Optical coherence tomography patterns of stent restenosis. Am Heart J. 2009;158:284–93.
17. van Soest G, Regar E, Goderie TP, Gonzalo N, Koljenović S, van Leenders GJ, et al. Pitfalls in plaque characterization by OCT: image artifacts in native coronary arteries. JACC Cardiovasc Imaging. 2011;4:810–3.

Acute Coronary Syndrome: Ruptured and Intact Fibrous Caps

2

2.1 Introduction

Coronary thrombosis is the most common cause of acute coronary syndromes (ACS), including sudden coronary death (SCD). Plaque rupture (PRU) in most cases, plaque erosion (PER) uncommonly, and calcified nodule (CaN) rarely have been demonstrated to be the main mechanisms underlying acute coronary thrombosis in both ex vivo and in vivo studies. In postmortem pathologic studies of subjects who died suddenly of coronary heart disease more than two thirds of the fatal events were related to PRU followed by thrombotic occlusion (Fig. 2.1). The acute coronary events were caused by thrombotic occlusion caused by PER (Fig. 2.2) in another third, and CaN was observed in 2–5% of cases [1–4]. Several clinical optical coherence tomography (OCT) studies have confirmed the autopsy data by establishing plaque rupture as the most frequent lesion identified in patients with ACS in vivo [5–10]. Patients with OCT erosion were younger, had a lower frequency of lipid plaque, a thicker fibrous cap, and less severe stenosis. They also presented less frequently with ST-segment elevation myocardial infarction (STEMI) than those with plaque rupture [7, 11]. A combined OCT and intravascular ultrasound (IVUS) study demonstrated that the incidence of PRU, PER, and CaN in 112 patients with acute STEMI was 64%, 27%, and 8%, respectively [9]. PER was characterized by fewer features of plaque vulnerability compared to PRU, including smaller plaque burden, lack of positive remodeling, and lipid richness. In the setting of ACS, high-resolution intravascular imaging with OCT can characterize plaque pathology at the time of intervention and allows better understanding of the etiology of STEMI. Acute events have been broadly classified as associated with ruptured fibrous cap (RFC) or intact fibrous cap (IFC) [12]. A recent OCT study of STEMI patients supports an alternative treatment strategy for patients with OCT-verified plaque erosion wherein nonobstructive lesions might be managed without stenting [13]. However, whether or not distinguishing among different plaque characteristics in STEMI patients undergoing percutaneous coronary intervention (PCI) can help develop personalized treatment strategies leading to improved long-term outcomes remains a matter of debate [14, 15]. Much more data are necessary to develop clinical guidelines regarding the role of OCT in the selection of therapy in patients with STEMI.

Spontaneous coronary artery dissection (SCAD) is a rare but important cause of ACS with an incidence of 0.1–2.1% as reported by angiographic and intravascular imaging studies [8, 9, 12, 16–18]. The majority of SCAD patients are young women manifesting ACS with no risk factors for atherosclerosis. Around a quarter of SCAD cases occurred either postpartum or with use of oral contraceptive [19]. Prompt diagnosis and treatment of patients with SCAD improve survival. The survival rate has been improved up to 95% as a result of advances in imaging modalities and therapy. Therapeutic options include medical therapy, percutaneous coronary intervention, and surgery. Thrombolysis is avoided in patients suspected of SCAD-related myocardial infarction. While diagnostic accuracy of angiography for SCAD is limited, OCT imaging can provide substantial insights into the morphologic features of the condition, including entry point, double lumen, and intramural hematoma [20, 21]. Small dissections or smooth stenoses mostly from an intramural hematoma may not be detected by coronary angiography; this leads to under-reporting of the phenomenon and underestimation the true prevalence of SCAD. Another cause of myocardial infarction in young patients less than 45 years old might be hypercoagulable states characterized by recurrent arterial and venous thrombosis [22]. However, this could be difficult to differentiate from PER. It can also be associated with other autoimmune diseases, for example, systemic lupus erythematosus (SLE). Patients with SLE have accelerated development of atherosclerosis as a result of nontraditional factors present in SLE

Electronic Supplementary Material The online version of this chapter (doi:10.1007/978-3-319-62666-6_2) contains supplementary material, which is available to authorized users.

A. Kini et al., *Atlas of Coronary Intravascular Optical Coherence Tomography*, DOI 10.1007/978-3-319-62666-6_2

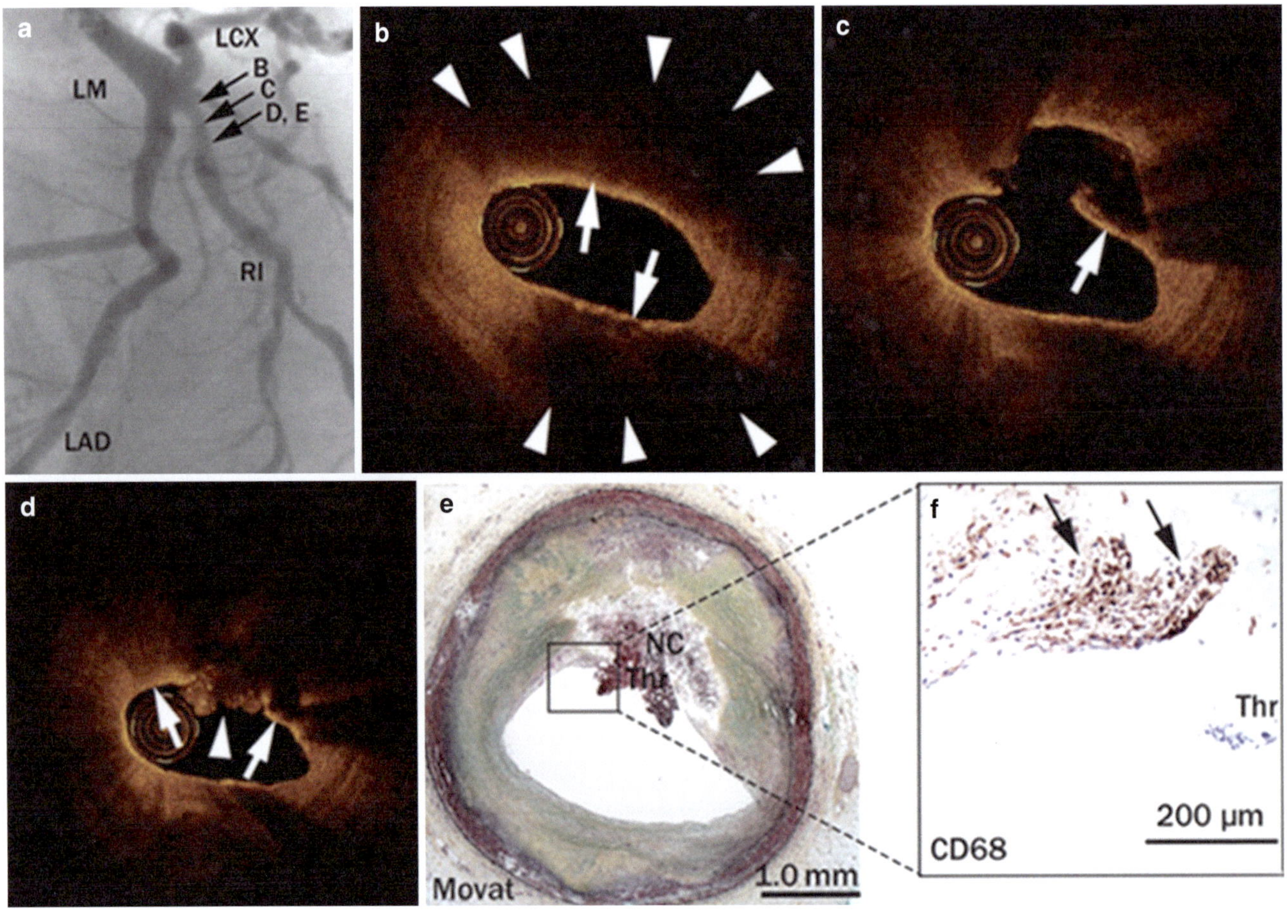

Fig. 2.1 A 45-year-old man with a history of hypertension, diabetes mellitus, and hyperlipidemia died suddenly after jogging during his lunch break. (**a**) Postmortem angiography showed mild luminal narrowing with haziness at proximal RI. (**b–d**) Serial OCT images revealed the presence of plaque rupture (in panels c and d) with a nonocclusive luminal thrombus (*white arrowhead* in **d**) and an adjacent distinct superficial signal-rich region (*white arrows* in panel **b**) with rapid attenuation (*white arrowheads* in **b**) indicating thin-cap fibroatheroma. A disrupted fibrous cap also shows a distinct superficial signal-rich region (*white arrows* in **c** and **d**). (**e**) Histologic examination confirmed the presence of plaque rupture with an acute fibrin-rich thrombus (shown as Thr) overlying the NC (section stained with movat pentachrome stain). (f) Immunostaining for CD68+ macrophages demonstrated substantial infiltration of macrophages within the disrupted fibrous cap (*black arrows*). *LAD* left anterior descending coronary artery, *LCX* left circumflex coronary artery, *LM* left main coronary artery, *NC* necrotic core, *OCT* optical coherence tomography; *RI* ramus intermedius. (*Reprinted from* Otsuka et al. [11]; with permission)

in addition to traditional risk factors, and they should be considered as high-risk patients for CAD [23].

Coronary spasm (CS) plays an important role in the pathogenesis of an acute coronary event [12, 24–27]. Because it is a transient phenomenon, morphologic features of CS culprit segments have not been fully understood. Most pathologic reports are case studies of patients presumed to have died from coronary vasospasm. Diagnosis is not always possible with coronary angiography alone. OCT allows detailed in vivo examination of the morphologic characteristics of coronary arteries in patients with CS [28–31]. Coronary segments affected by CS are characterized by diffuse intimal thickening without lipid or calcium accumulation. An additional OCT feature of intima-media separation from adventitia was observed in some CS cases [30, 31].

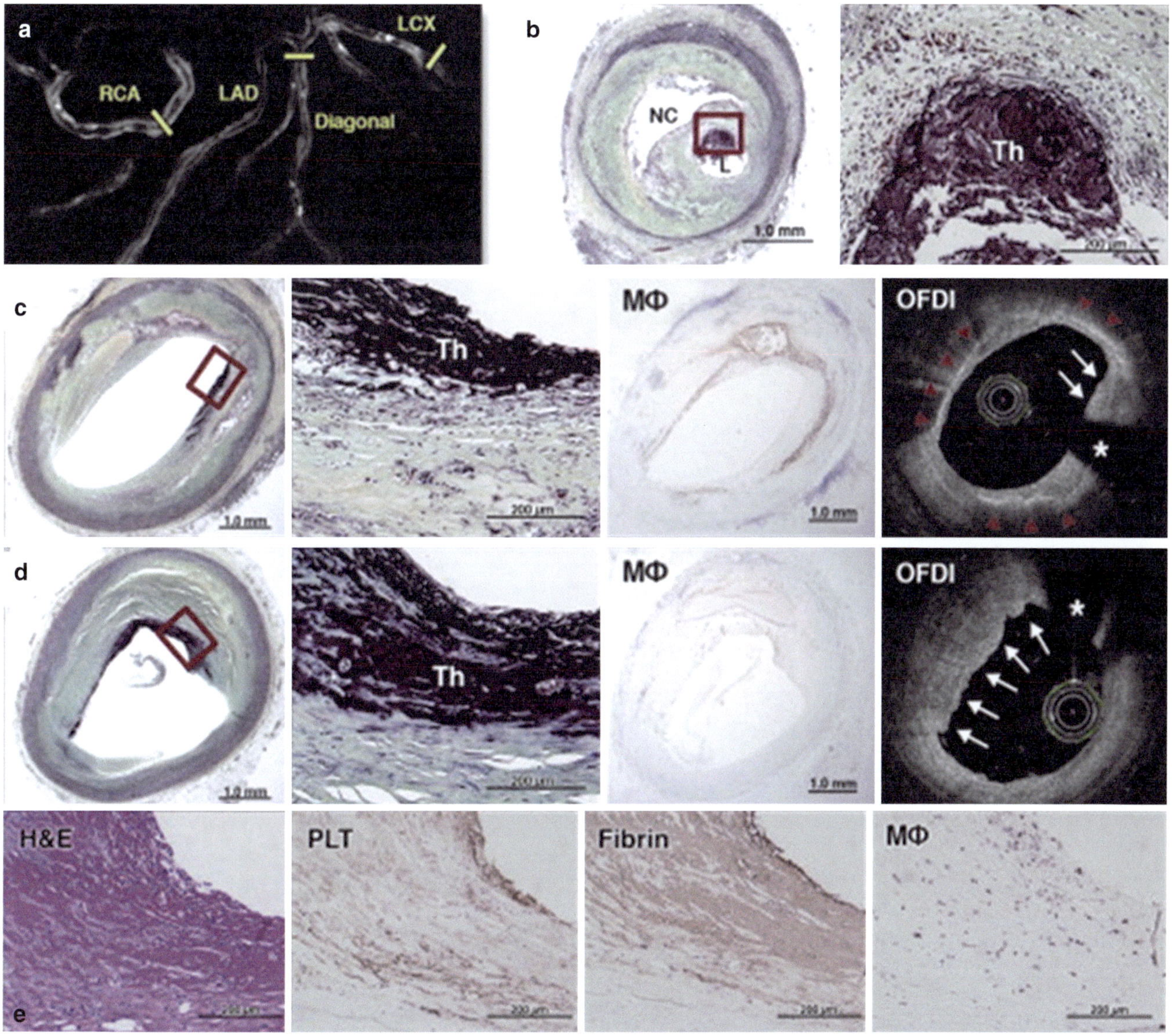

Fig. 2.2 Multiple plaque erosions in three major coronary arteries. (**a**) Postmortem radiography showed focal mild calcification in all major coronary arteries. (**b**) Histologic examination showed the LCX with a nonocclusive platelet-rich organizing thrombus (Th) with underlying late fibroatheroma. (**c**) The right coronary artery (RCA) showed a luminal fibrin-rich organizing thrombus with an underlying late fibroatheroma. (**d**) The diagonal branch artery also showed a luminal fibrin-rich organizing thrombus with an underlying pathologic intimal thickening. Fibrin-rich thrombi with a few inflammatory cells are seen on the luminal surface. Corresponding macrophage (MΦ) stain and optical frequency domain imaging images (OFDI) (Terumo; Tokyo, Japan) are depicted. Moderate macrophage infiltration is seen around the circumference of the vessel (*red arrows*); however, the culprit site (*white arrows*) is devoid of macrophages in the RCA. Note the absence of macrophage in the diagonal branch (macrophages stained section of **d**). OFDI showed luminal surface irregularity with minimal attenuation because the thrombus had focal areas of platelets interspersed with large areas of fibrin in the RCA and the diagonal branch (*white arrows*). A bright layer with attenuation (*red arrowheads*) indicates the presence of macrophages in RCA (**c**). (**e**) Serial sections at high power stained by hematoxylin and eosin (H&E), platelet ([PLT] CD61), fibrin (fibrin II), and macrophage (CD68) stained images from the box in d are shown. Platelet stains (*brown*) show few superficial and interspersed platelets with a predominance of fibrin (*brown*, *adjacent section*) and rare macrophage infiltration (*brown*). *Asterisk* indicates placement of guidewire. *L* lumen, *LAD* left anterior descending, *NC* necrotic core. (*Reprinted from* Yahagi et al. [32]; with permisison)

2.2 Case 1. Non-ST-Elevation Myocardial Infarction – Thin Cap: Going, Going, Gone... (Figs. 2.3, 2.4 and Video 2.1)

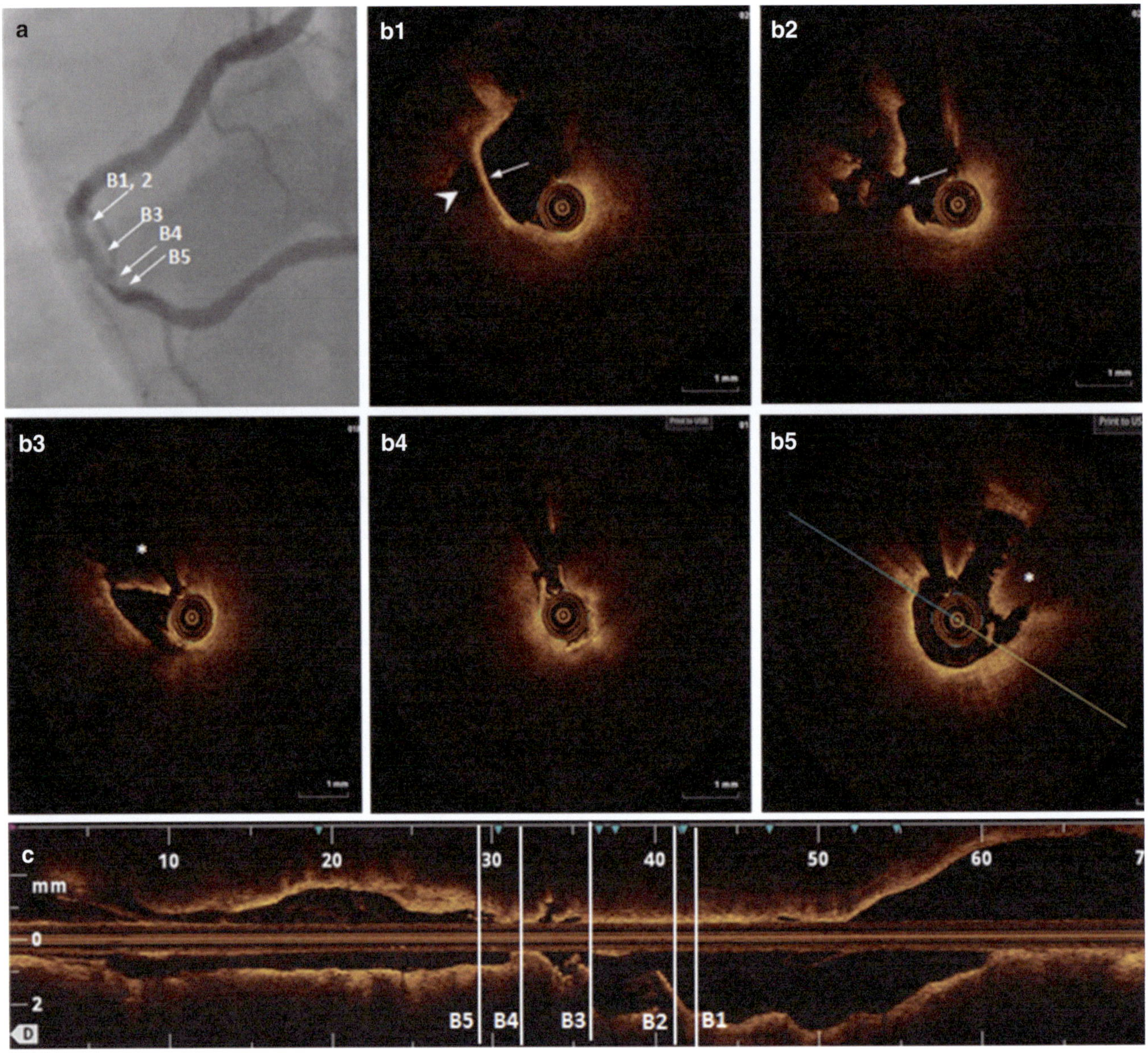

Fig. 2.3 Coronary angiography and OCT imaging before PCI. A 49-year-old male, an ex-smoker with a history of prior myocardial infarction, hyperlipidemia, controlled hypertension, and diet-controlled diabetes presented with a non-ST-elevation myocardial infarction (NSTEMI). Cardiac enzymes (cTnI 8.68 ng/mL) were elevated, and a small apical thrombus was identified by echocardiography. Coronary angiography showed a 90–95% stenosis with a filling defect in the distal RCA (**a**). OCT imaging of the segment revealed the presence of plaque rupture (**b2**, *arrow*) proximal to the site of the minimal lumen area (MLA) (**b4**). An intact thin fibrous cap (*arrow*) overlying a ruptured plaque cavity (*arrowhead*) was visualized proximal to the site of rupture (**b1**). In addition, large red thrombi were detected by OCT proximal (**b3**, *asterisk*) and distal (**b5**, *asterisk*) to MLA

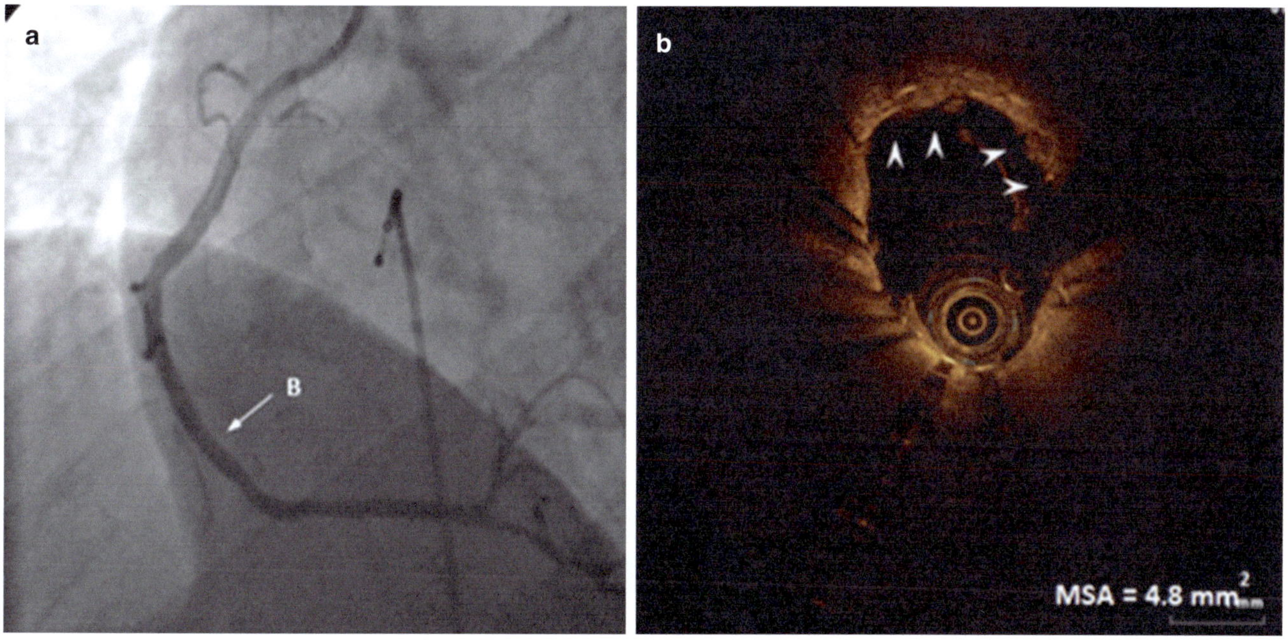

Fig. 2.4 Coronary angiography and OCT imaging after PCI. An everolimus eluting stent (3.5/28 mm) was implanted successfully in the culprit lesion (**a**). Post-stent OCT pullback confirmed a satisfactory apposition and expansion of the stent with minimal stent area (MSA) of 4.8 mm^2 (**b**). Small tissue protrusions were detected at the site of MSA (**b**, *arrowheads*). Based on pre-intervention OCT findings, acute plaque rupture was identified as an underlying mechanism for ACS in the case, while post-stenting OCT was used to confirm optimal stent expansion and apposition

2.3 Case 2. Plaque Rupture in Unstable Angina Pectoris: Subcritical Stenosis, Plaque Rupture, and Acute Event (Figs. 2.5 and 2.6, Videos 2.2 and 2.3)

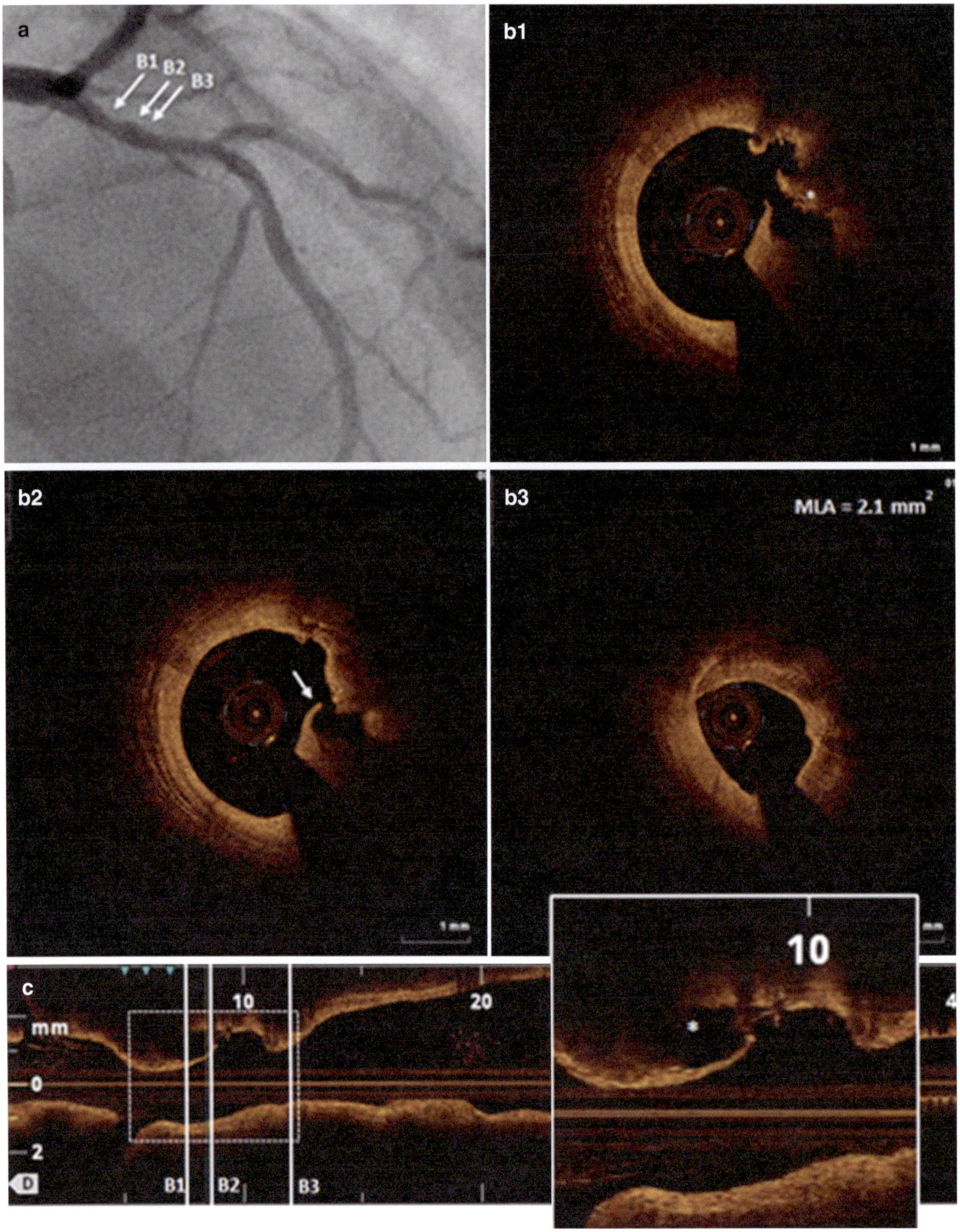

Fig. 2.5 A 53-year-old male, a smoker with a history of hyperlipidemia presented to the emergency room with severe angina at rest. A coronary angiogram revealed 50–60% stenosis in the proximal left anterior descending artery (LAD) (**a**). OCT pullback performed in the LAD detected a fibrous cap rupture (**b2**, *arrow*) distal to the site of the MLA (**b3**). A large cavity associated with plaque rupture can be visualized in the longitudinal OCT image **c** (*inset, asterisk*). A nonocclusive red luminal thrombus was detected distal to the site of rupture (**b1**, *asterisk*), demonstrating that PRU in subcritically occluded vessels may result in unstable angina

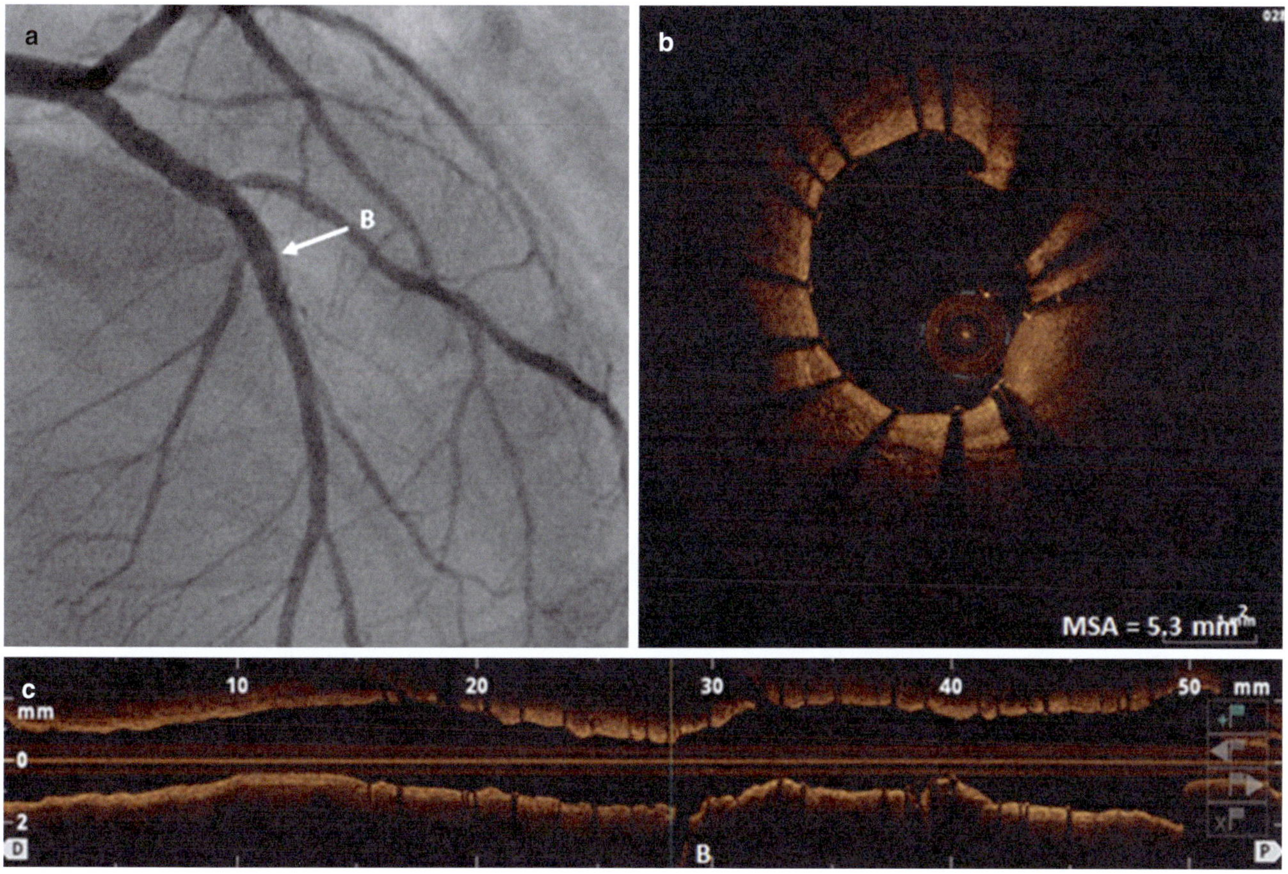

Fig. 2.6 Coronary angiography and OCT after PCI. A 3.25/33 mm everolimus eluting coronary stent was successfully implanted in the proximal LAD (**a**). Good apposition and expansion of the LAD stent were confirmed by post-PCI OCT pullback (**b**, **c**). In this case, OCT imaging of the culprit lesion helped clarify the etiology of ACS as acute rupture of vulnerable atherosclerotic plaque and verify the optimal stent placement

2.4 Case 3. ST-Elevation Myocardial Infarction Caused by Plaque Rupture and Total Occlusion of the LAD: An Accident with a Traffic Jam Ahead (Figs. 2.7 and 2.8, Videos 2.4 and 2.5)

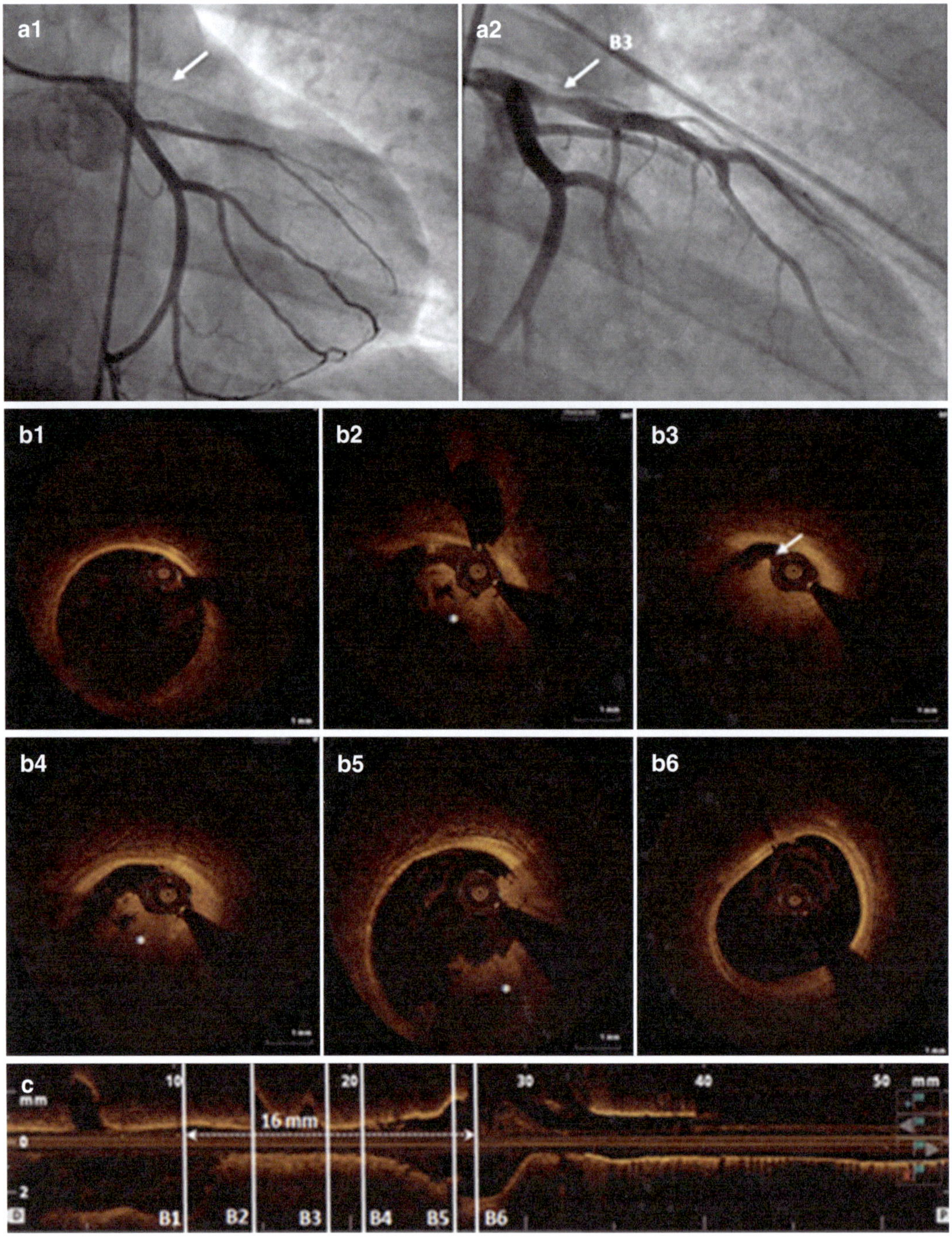

Fig. 2.7 A 33-year-old male who was a former smoker with hyperlipidemia and a family history of CAD presented at the emergency room with substernal chest pain at rest, which started 10 min after exercise. An electrocardiogram showed anterior wall ST-elevation myocardial infarction (STEMI). A coronary angiogram demonstrated total thrombotic occlusion of the proximal LAD (**a1**). By means of a thrombectomy with multiple passages across the lesion, a large thrombus load was removed and anterograde flow was restored (**a2**). OCT imaging performed after thrombus aspiration detected a large irregular red thrombus still occupying the vessel lumen (**b2**, **b4**, **b5** *asterisk*). The residual thrombus prevented the identification of underlying vessel wall structures in the majority of OCT cross-sectional images, but a possible site of fibrous cap disruption was visualized in a few adjacent frames (**b3**, *arrow*), suggesting plaque rupture as the underlying mechanism of ACS in this case. Cross-sections with the largest lumen and least plaque in the segment were identified as distal (**b1**) and proximal (**b6**) references and landing zones for stenting. The mean reference lumen diameters were 4.3 mm for proximal reference and 4.7 mm for distal reference

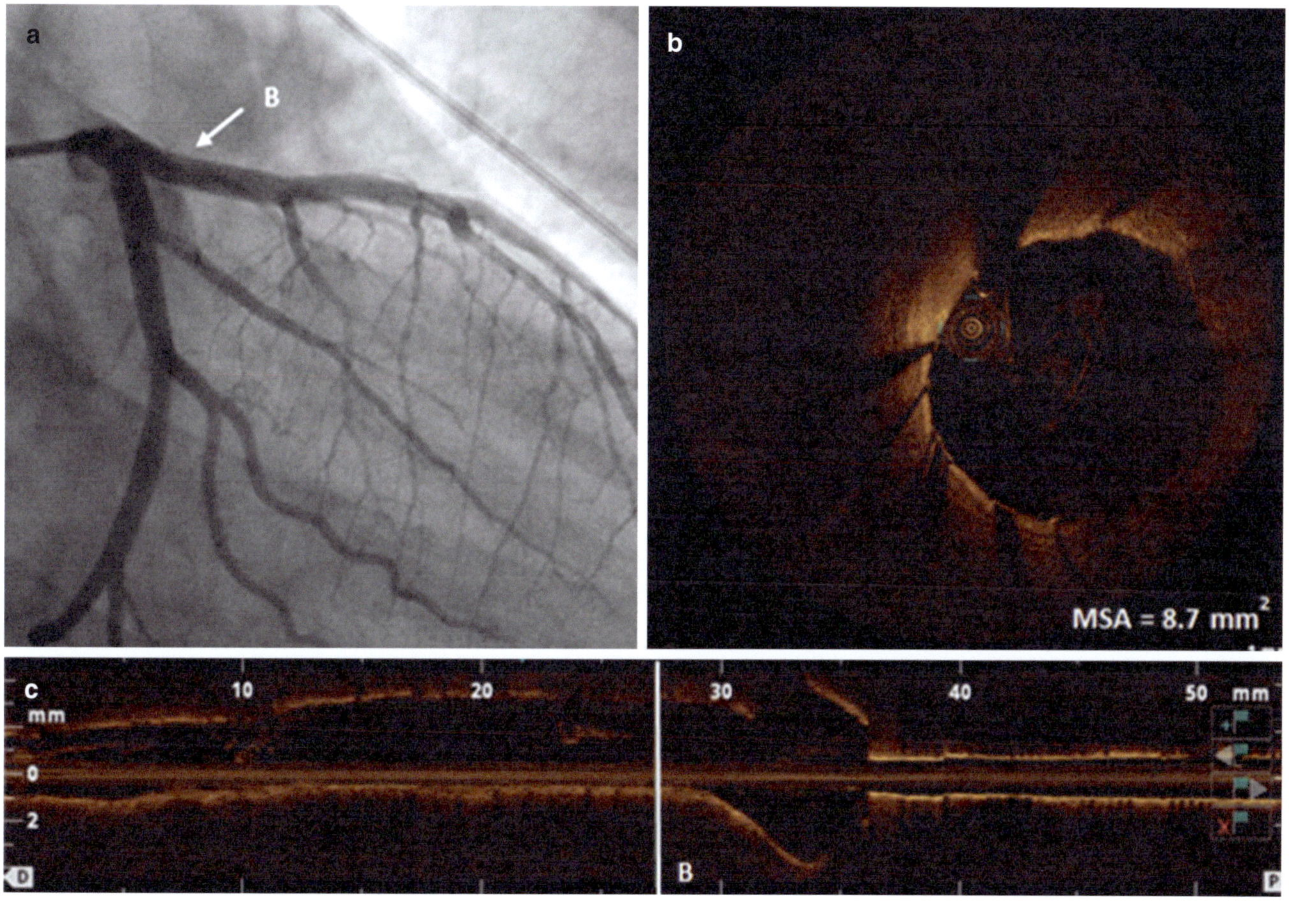

Fig. 2.8 Based on pre-PCI lesion assessment by OCT, a 4/15 mm everolimus eluting stent was selected for the lesion. A final post-stenting angiogram demonstrated satisfactory luminal gain at the proximal LAD (**a**). Good stent apposition and expansion with a minimal stent area of 8.7 mm^2 was shown by OCT (**b**, **c**). In this case, OCT imaging not only helped identify the pathophysiologic substrate of STEMI and to assess the extent of residual thrombus after thrombectomy but also facilitated stent sizing based on identification of proximal and distal landing zones

2.5 Case 4. ST-Elevation Myocardial Infarction Arising from Plaque Erosion: Acute Coronary Event with Intact Fibrous Cap (Figs. 2.9 and 2.10, Video 2.6)

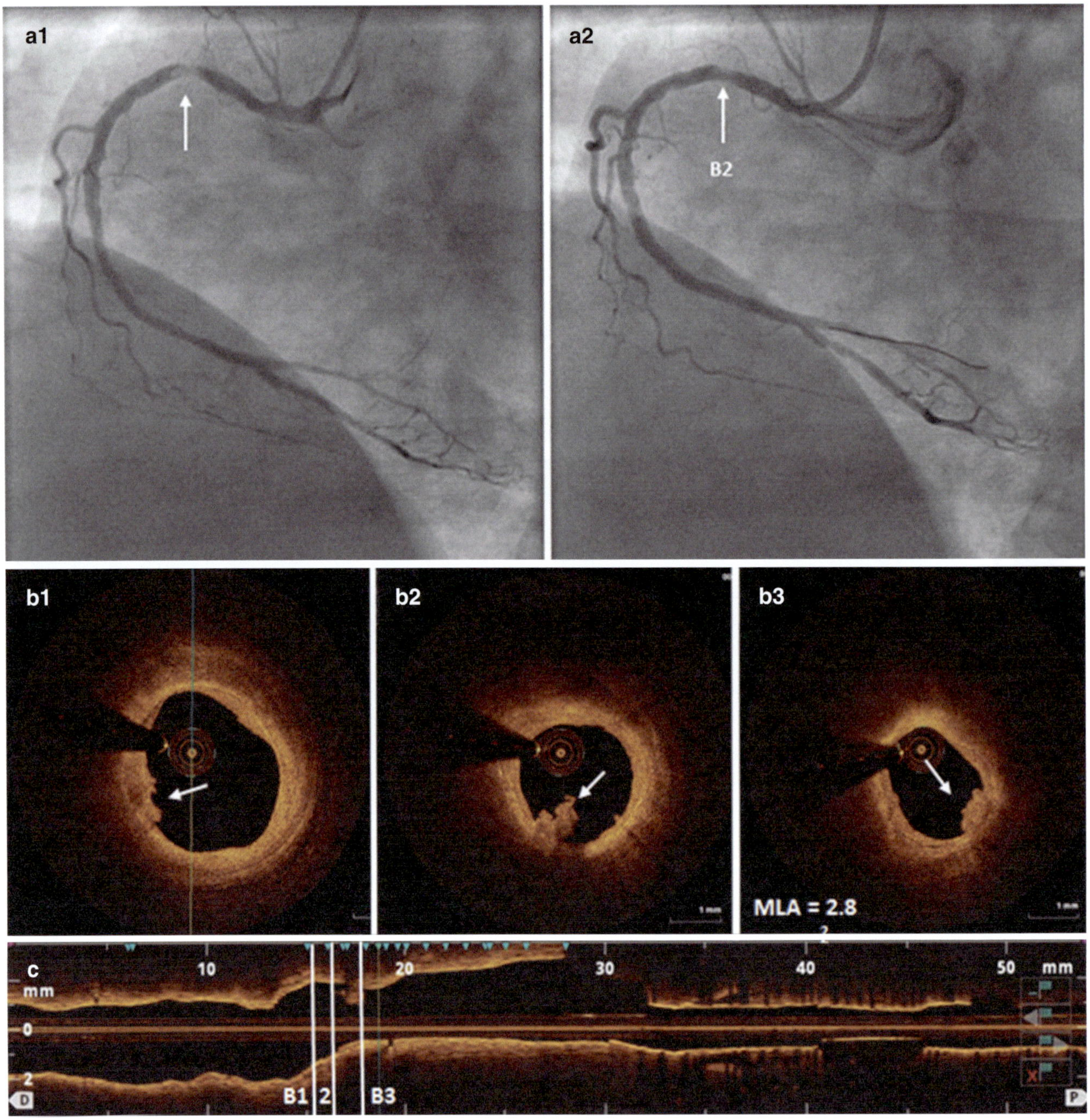

Fig. 2.9 A 51-year-old female with uncontrolled hypertension and deep vein thrombosis (DVT) presented with substernal chest pain (CCS class IV angina). The ECG showed ST-elevation in leads II, III, and aVF. Emergency coronary angiography showed subtotal occlusion of the proximal RCA (**a1**, *arrow*). A coronary angiogram after thrombectomy with multiple passages across the lesion showed a partial resolution of the intraluminal filling defect (**a2**). Post-thrombectomy OCT acquisition of the corresponding segment detected an obstructive lesion with an MLA of 2.8 mm^2 (**b3**) and demonstrated the presence of a signal-rich irregular mass protruding into the lumen. In contrast to the mass shown in Figs. 2.1 and 2.3, this case mass is characterized by mild signal attenuation and easily delineated borders, suggesting a white thrombus (**b1**–**b3**, *arrows*). The underlying vessel structures are not obscured as in the previous examples of red thrombus, which allows a frame by frame examination of the lesion. The examination did not find evidence of plaque rupture or a large lipid core, suggesting fibrous cap erosion as the mechanism responsible for the ACS. Because of the presence of significant stenosis, the lesion was treated with an everolimus-eluting platinum chromium stent (3.5/12 mm) implantation

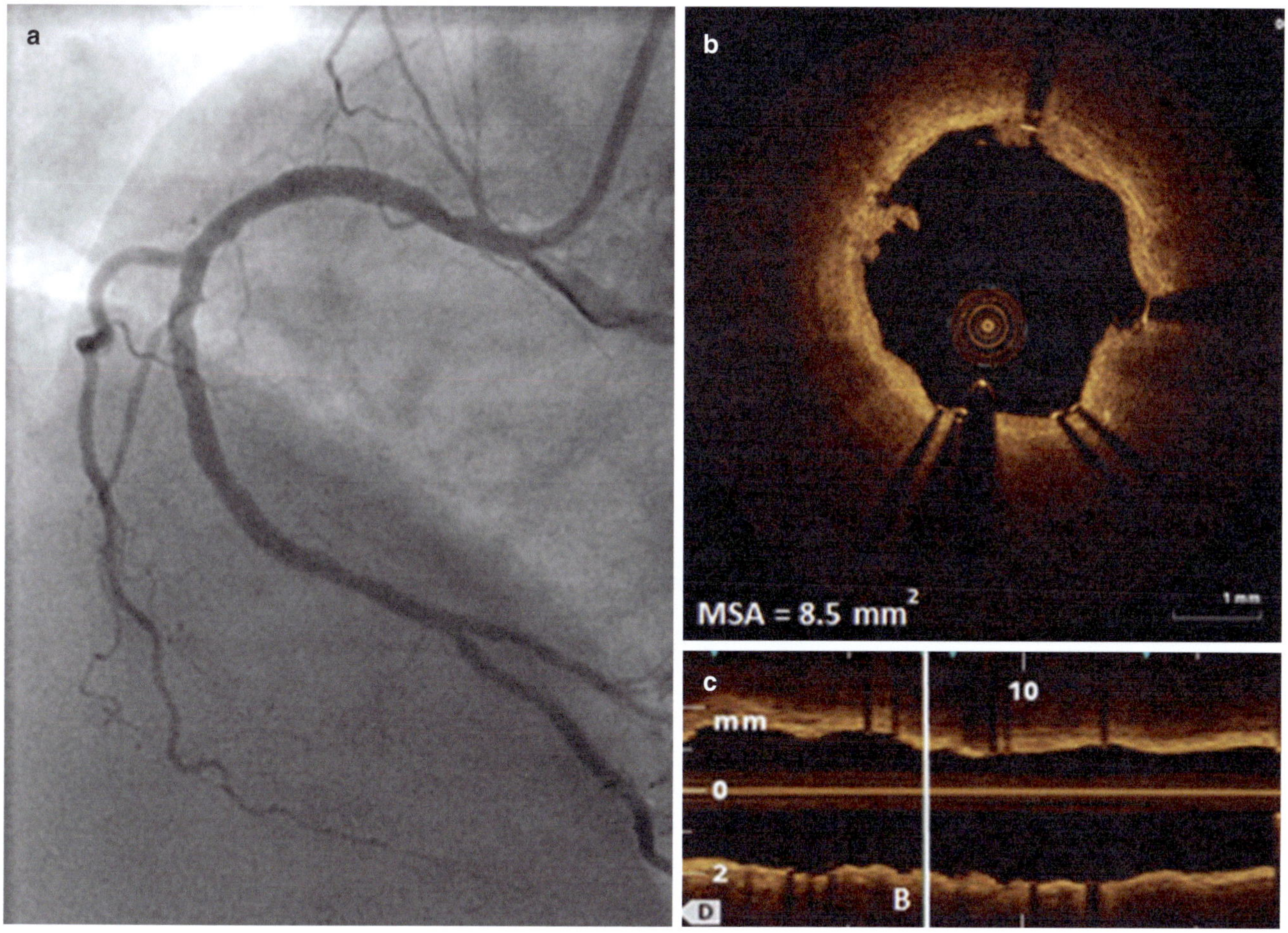

Fig. 2.10 A final post-PCI coronary angiogram showed successful stent deployment in the proximal RCA (**a**), which was verified by an OCT pullback. There was no strut malapposition detected by OCT, and the stent was well expanded with a minimal area of 8.5 mm^2 (**b**)

2.6 Case 5. Multimodality Imaging of Plaque Erosion in Non-ST-Elevation Myocardial Infarction: A Young Woman Who Smokes May Be Vulnerable (Figs. 2.11 and 2.12, Video 2.7)

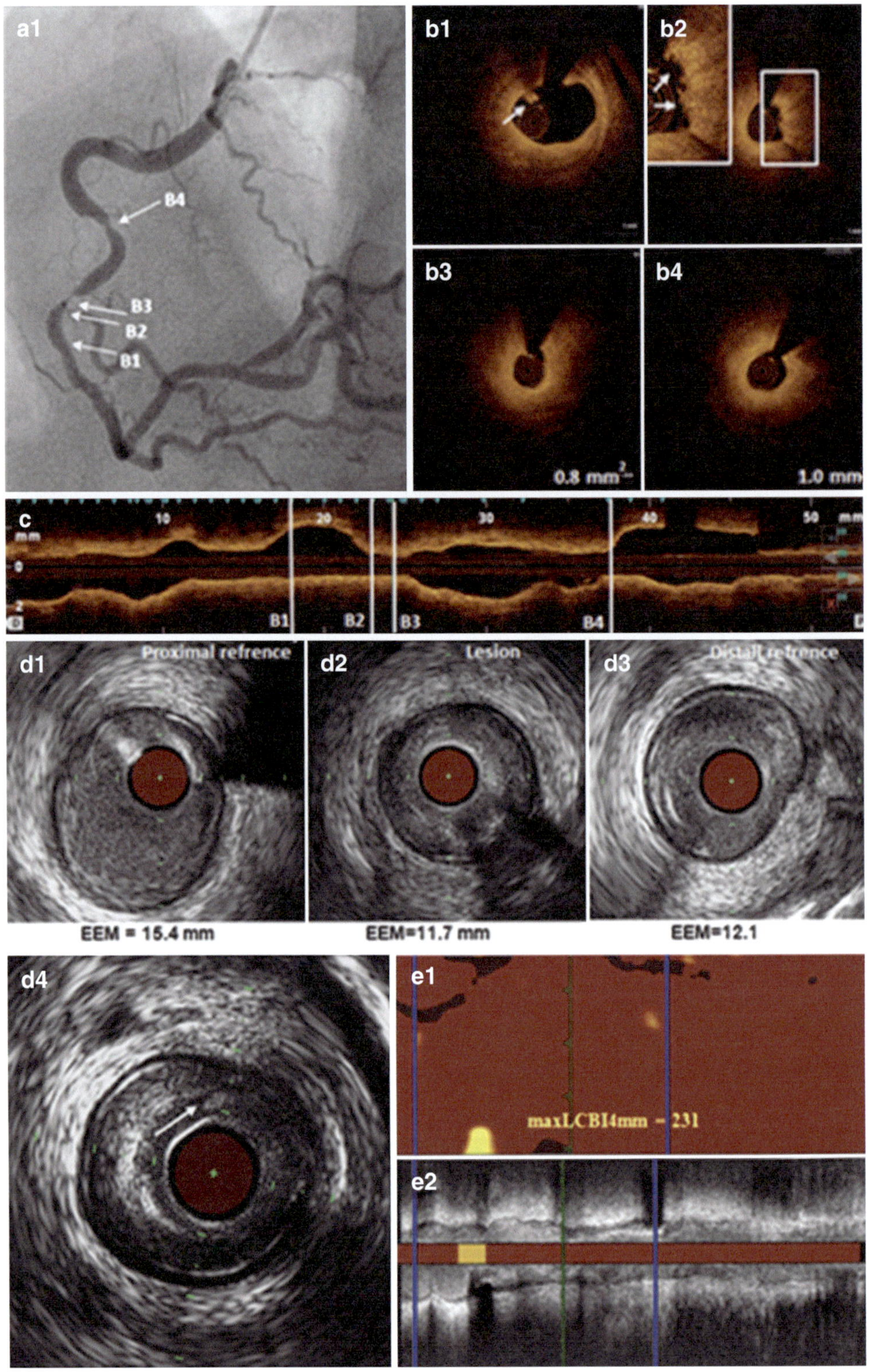

Fig. 2.11 A 40-year-old female with a history of controlled hypertension, smoking, rheumatoid arthritis, and substance abuse presented with NSTEMI (cTnI peak 7.7 ng/ml). Coronary angiography demonstrated a 70–80% stenosis in the proximal and 90–95% obstruction in the mid RCA (**a1**). OCT pullback showed two fibrotic plaques with an MLA of 1.0 and 0.8 mm^2, respectively (**b4**, **b3**), and several small while thrombi distal to the middle RCA lesion (**b1**, **b2**, *arrows*). Serial OCT cross-sectional images of the culprit lesions did not detect plaque rupture; however, an irregular lumen surface was visualized with an attached mural thrombus (*arrows*) overlying a fibrous plaque (**b2**) consistent with plaque erosion. In addition to OCT pullback, combined intravascular ultrasound (IVUS) and near infrared spectroscopy (NIRS) imaging were performed. Pre-PCI IVUS (**d1**–**d4**) and NIRS (**e1**, **e2**) images of RCA showed a negatively remodeled fibrotic plaque with a remodeling index 0.85 and an MLA of 1.6 mm^2 (**d2**, *green lines in* **e1**, **e2**). The remodeling index (RI) was calculated using the mean of the proximal (**d1**) and distal (**d3**) external elastic membrane (EEM) cross-sectional area (CSA) measurements shown for each frame; blue lines in **e1** and **e2** indicate proximal and distal references. A small intraluminal thrombus detected by OCT (**b1**) is shown in the corresponding IVUS cross-sectional image (**d4**, *arrow*). OCT allows clearer thrombus visualization owing to its higher resolution. In this case, OCT findings suggested that the etiology of ACS originates from the erosion of an unstable plaque

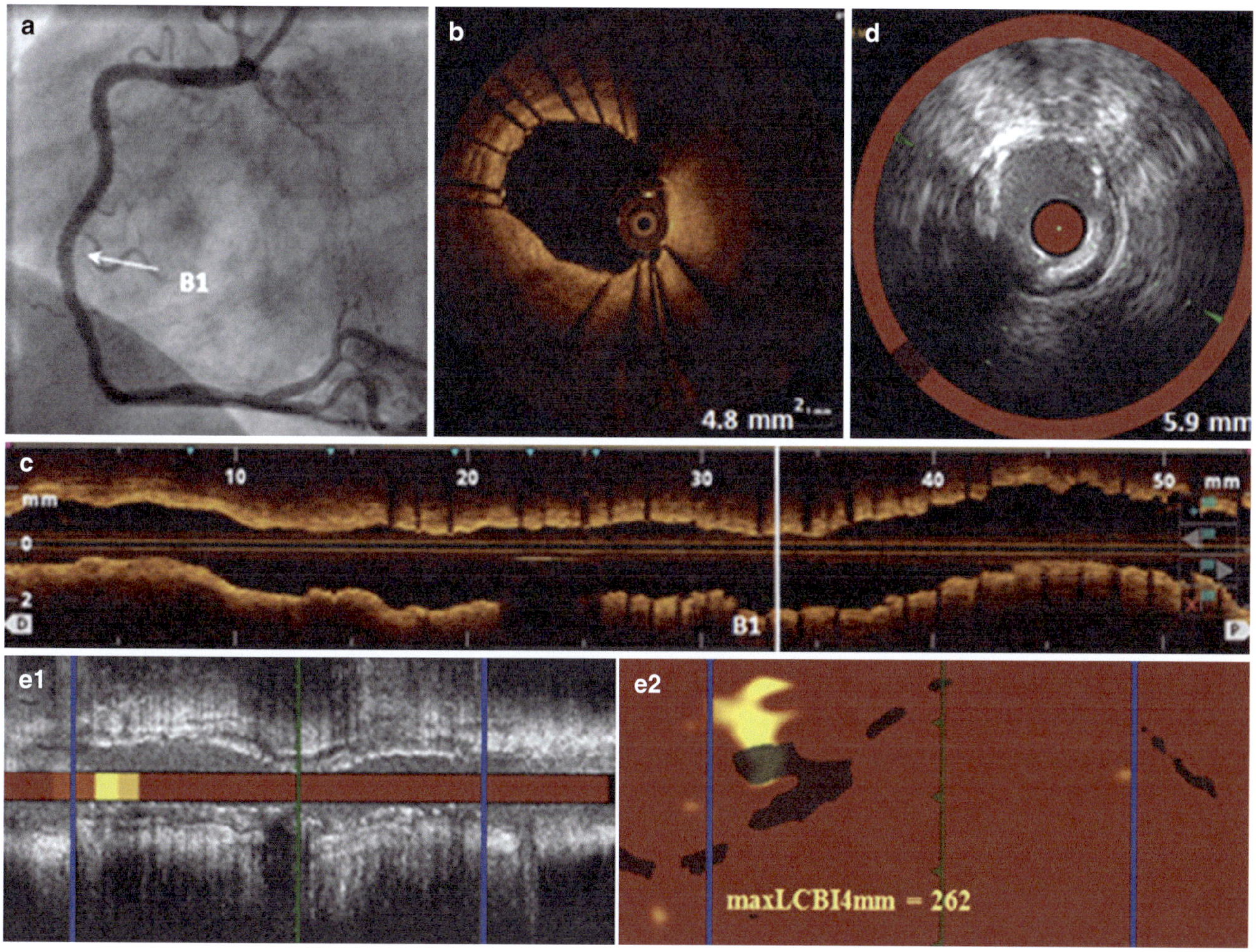

Fig. 2.12 Post-stent angiogram, OCT, and IVUS/NIRS images. A 3/38-mm everolimus eluting stent was implanted to cover both proximal and mid RCA lesions (**a**). Post-stent intravascular imaging showed a well expanded and apposed stent with an MSA of 4.8 mm² by OCT (**b1**, **c**) and 5.9 mm² by IVUS (**d1**)*. Blue lines in **e1** and **e2** indicate the proximal and distal edges of the stent; the *green line* corresponds to the MSA site (**b**, **d**)

2.7 Case 6. Probable Plaque Erosion in Non-ST-Elevation Myocardial Infarction: Obviating a Need for a Stent in Plaque Erosion (Fig. 2.13, Video 2.8)

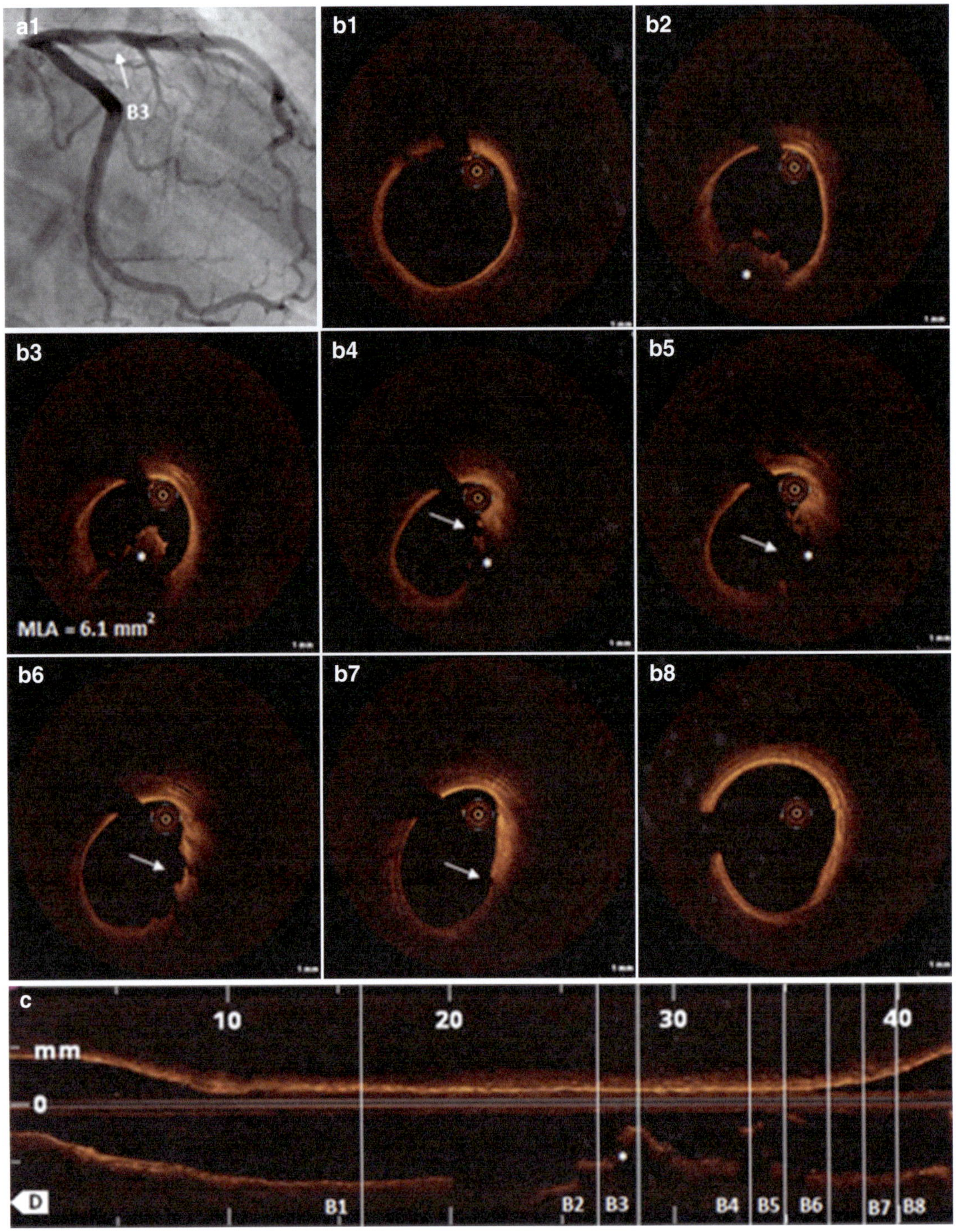

Fig. 2.13 Coronary angiography and OCT of proximal LAD before stenting. A 49-year-old male without a cardiac history presented with NSTEMI. The angiographic image showed a 30–50% moderate thrombotic lesion in the proximal LAD (**a1**), and OCT assessment confirmed nonobstructive stenosis with a minimal lumen area of 6.1 mm^2. Because of the presence of a large red thrombus (**b2**–**b5**, C, *asterisks*), the underlying plaque morphology was not visualized well by OCT imaging. A series of OCT cross-sectional images from the proximal to the distal reference of the culprit lesion (**b1**–**b8**) failed to demonstrate a detectable site of plaque rupture. Initially, a possible rupture site was suspected in frames **b4**–**b7** (*arrow*). However, the feature was classified as a tangential artifact after taking into account the OCT catheter position with respect to the vessel wall and the presence of the feature in the proximal frame with minimal plaque (**b7**, *arrow*). There was also no lipid or calcium accumulation immediately proximal or distal to the site of the thrombus. Taken together, the OCT findings suggested a case of probable OCT erosion [7]. Based on the findings, the patient was discharged on maximal medical therapy without stent implantation

2.8 Case 7. Unstable Angina in a Young Patient with Systemic Lupus Erythematosus (Figs. 2.14 and 2.15, Video 2.9)

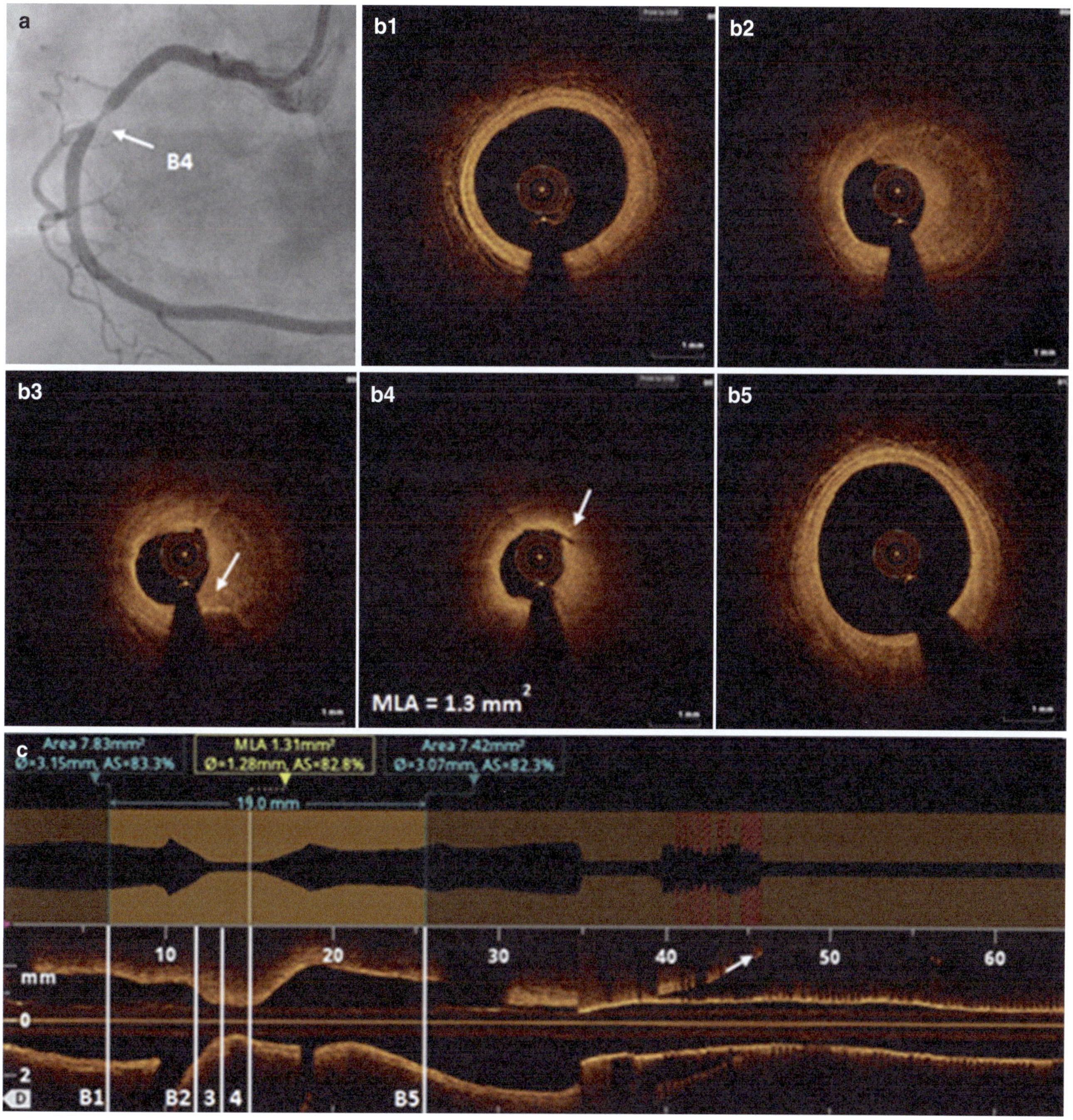

Fig. 2.14 Coronary angiography and OCT of the RCA before PCI. A 34-year-old female with systemic lupus erythematosus (SLE) and a history of proximal LAD STEMI 3 years earlier presented with chest pain on minimal exertion and at rest. While her proximal LAD stent was patent, a coronary angiogram showed a severe 90–95% focal stenosis of the RCA (**a**). OCT imaging performed after lesion predilatation revealed a large homogeneous mostly fibrous plaque (**b1**, **b2**) with macrophage accumulation observed in several adjacent frames (**b3**, *arrow*). The minimal lumen area was 1.3 mm² and the lumen area stenosis was 82.8% based on automatic lumen profile assessment with distal and proximal references selected at frames **b1** and **b5**. The mean reference diameters were 3.15 and 3.07 mm at the distal and proximal reference sites. Based on the measurements, a 3.25/15 mm DES was selected for the lesion. A small intimal tear observed in several frames (**b4**, *arrow*) most probably resulted from predilatation

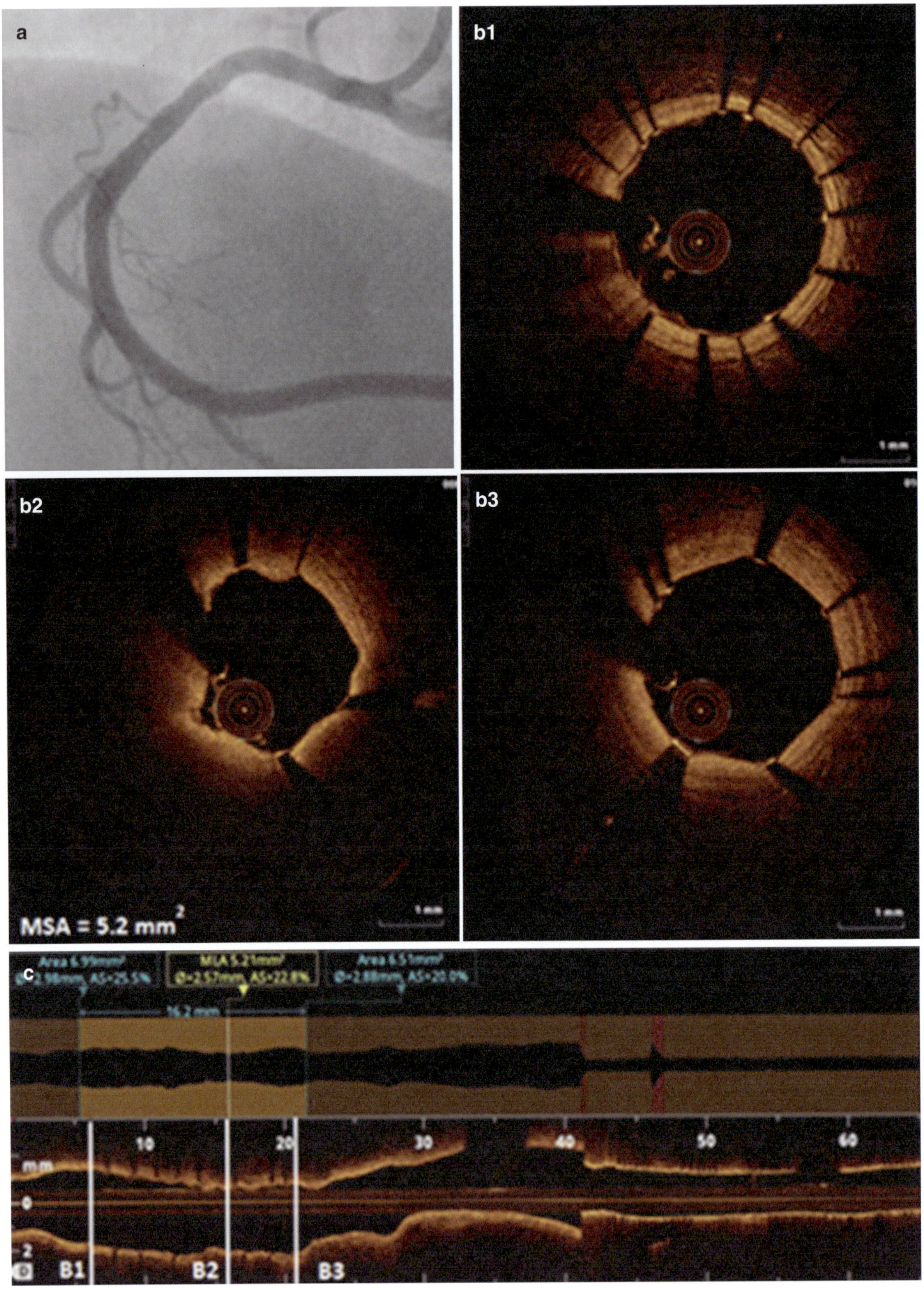

Fig. 2.15 Final poststenting angiography showed successful stent deployment in the RCA (**a**). OCT imaging confirmed optimal stent apposition and expansion with an MSA of 5.2 mm^2 (**b1**–**b3**, **c**). In this case of ACS in a young adult with SLE, OCT allowed characterization of the pathophysiology of the coronary event and guided intervention for selection of the best treatment strategy for the patient

2.9 Case 8. Spontaneous Coronary Vasospasm: Imaged, Verified, and Left Alone (Fig. 2.16, Video 2.10)

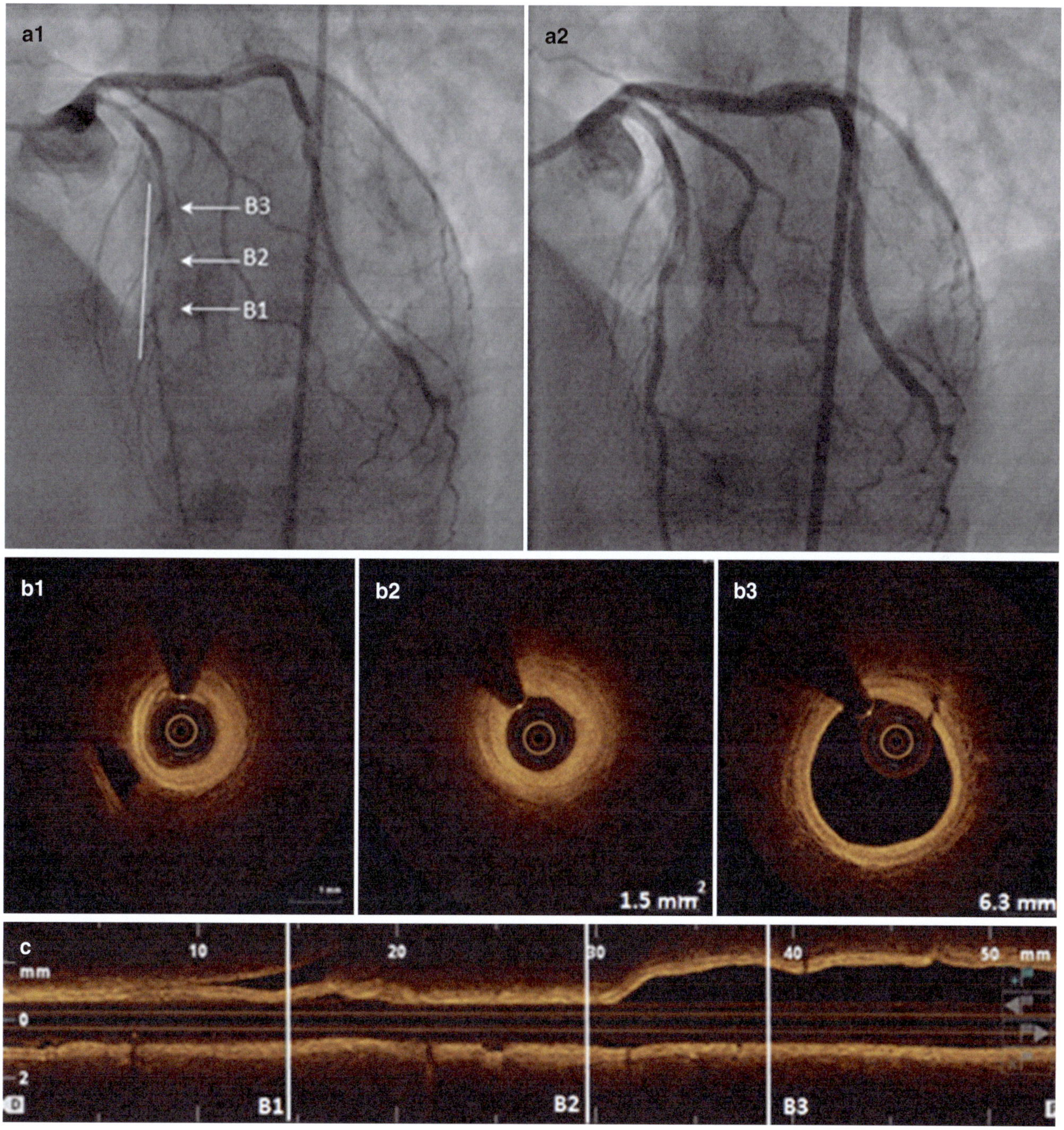

Fig. 2.16 Angiographic and OCT assessment of coronary spasm. A 61-year-old female with controlled hypertension, hyperlipidemia, and obesity presented at the Emergency Room with chest pain and shortness of breath at rest in a setting of NSTEMI (cTnI 2.8 ng/ml). A coronary angiogram of LAD demonstrated diffuse luminal narrowing with particularly severe stenosis in mid LAD (**a1**). OCT images demonstrated diffuse intimal thickening at the site of MLA of 1.5 mm^2 (**b2**) and distal to MLA (**b1**). The segment proximal to the MLA site demonstrated normal vessel anatomy (**b3**). No OCT evidence of plaque rupture or erosion was found. Vascular contraction disappeared after intracoronary injection of nitroglycerin (**a2**). Based on the findings, the main mechanism for ACS in this case was considered to be coronary vasospasm, and stent implantation was not required

2.10 Case 9. Postpartum Spontaneous Coronary Artery Dissection: *quod erat demonstrandum* (Figs. 2.17 and 2.18, Videos 2.11 and 2.12)

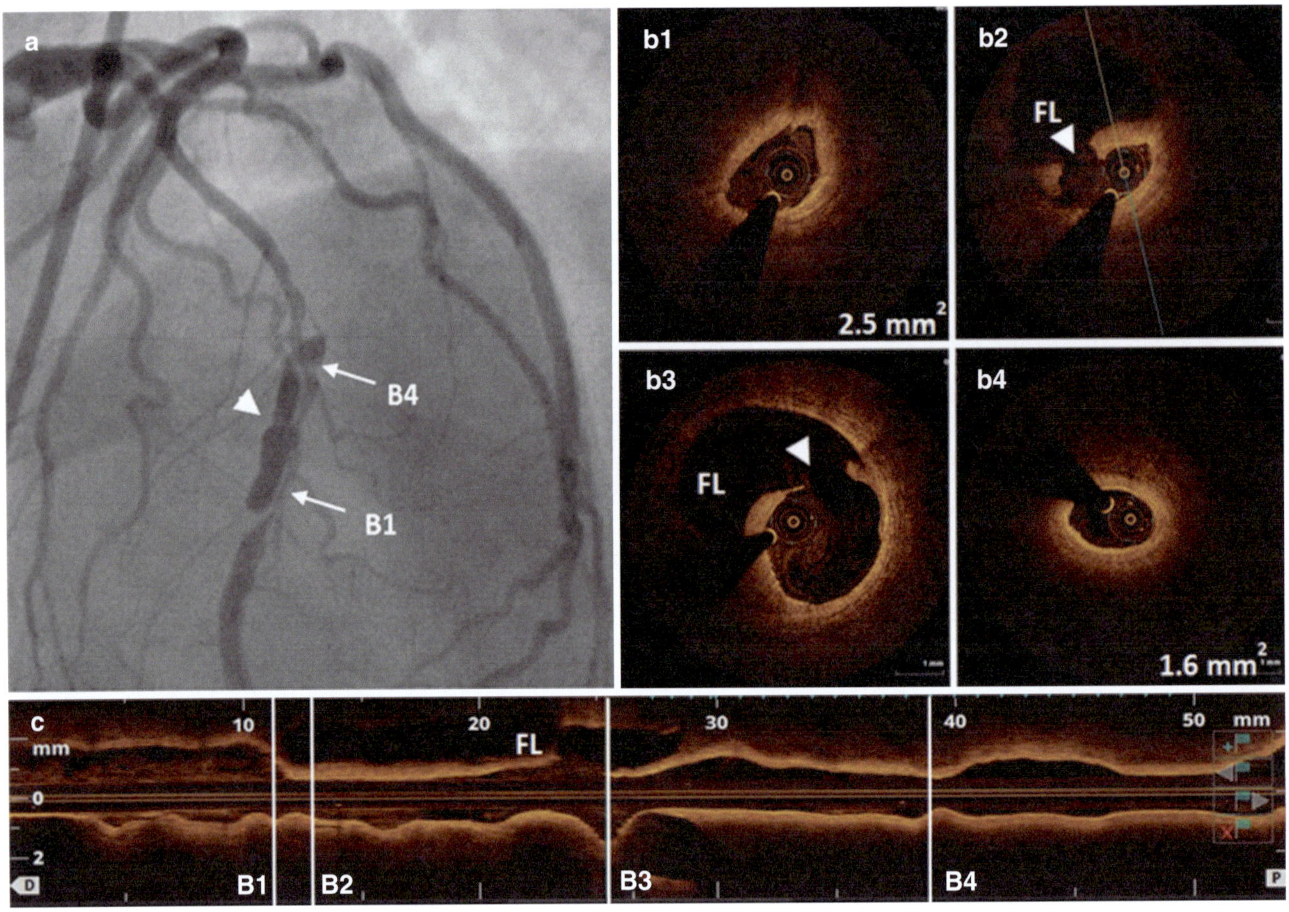

Fig. 2.17 Pre-PCI coronary angiography and OCT images. A 34-year-old female presented at a peripheral hospital with chest pain 7 days after caesarean section with bleeding complications. She had elevated troponin I and her EKG showed ST-elevation myocardial infarction. A spontaneous dissection of the LAD was revealed by coronary angiogram, and the patient was treated conservatively in the peripheral hospital. Over several following days she showed worsening of ischemic symptoms and was transferred for further management. A coronary angiogram confirmed the presence of spontaneous coronary artery dissection (SCAD) characterized by a double-lumen appearance (**a**, *arrowhead*) and a severe (90–95%) narrowing distal to the dissection (**a**, *arrow*). OCT imaging revealed a 19-mm false lumen (FL) (**c**) with entry and reentry sites shown by *arrowheads* in parts **b3** and **b2** correspondingly. Since two severe stenoses were detected proximal (**b4**) and distal (**b1**) to the dissection segment by OCT, a decision to treat the lesion with stent implantation was made by the operator

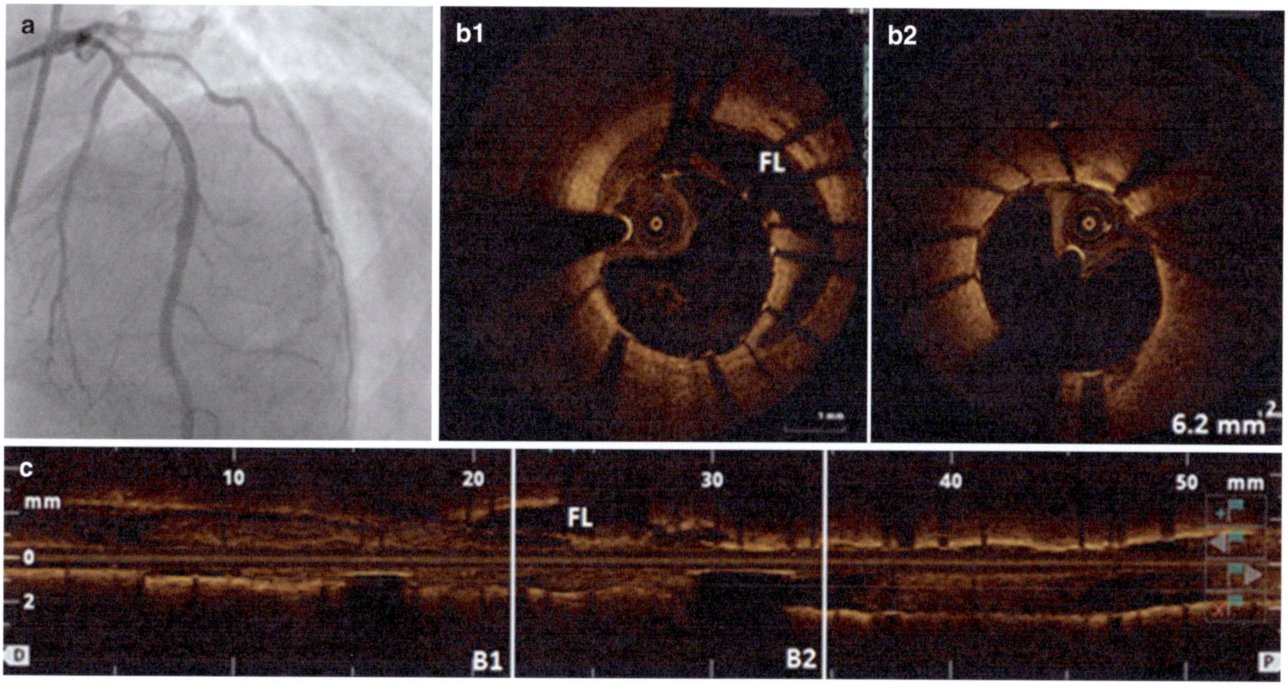

Fig. 2.18 Coronary angiogram and OCT after stenting. Two DES (3/38 mm and 3/18 mm) were successfully implanted in the mid LAD with good angiographic result (**a**). OCT confirmed that stent placement relieved the true lumen obstruction by sealing the false lumen, which resulted in a minimal stent area of 6.2 mm^2. Good stent apposition and expansion were observed in most of the stented segment; however, OCT visualized a 10-mm residual FL (**b1**, **c**). After intervention, patient made a full recovery and remained asymptomatic at 1 month follow-up. In this case of pregnancy-related SCAD, OCT imaging confirmed angiographically diagnosed SCAD and characterized its morphologic features. Based on OCT findings and increasing ischemic symptoms of the patient, interventional treatment was selected in this case

2.11 Case 10. Coronary Intramural Hematoma in Unstable Angina Pectoris: Another Example of an Acute Coronary Event with an Intact Fibrous Cap (Fig. 2.19, Video 2.13)

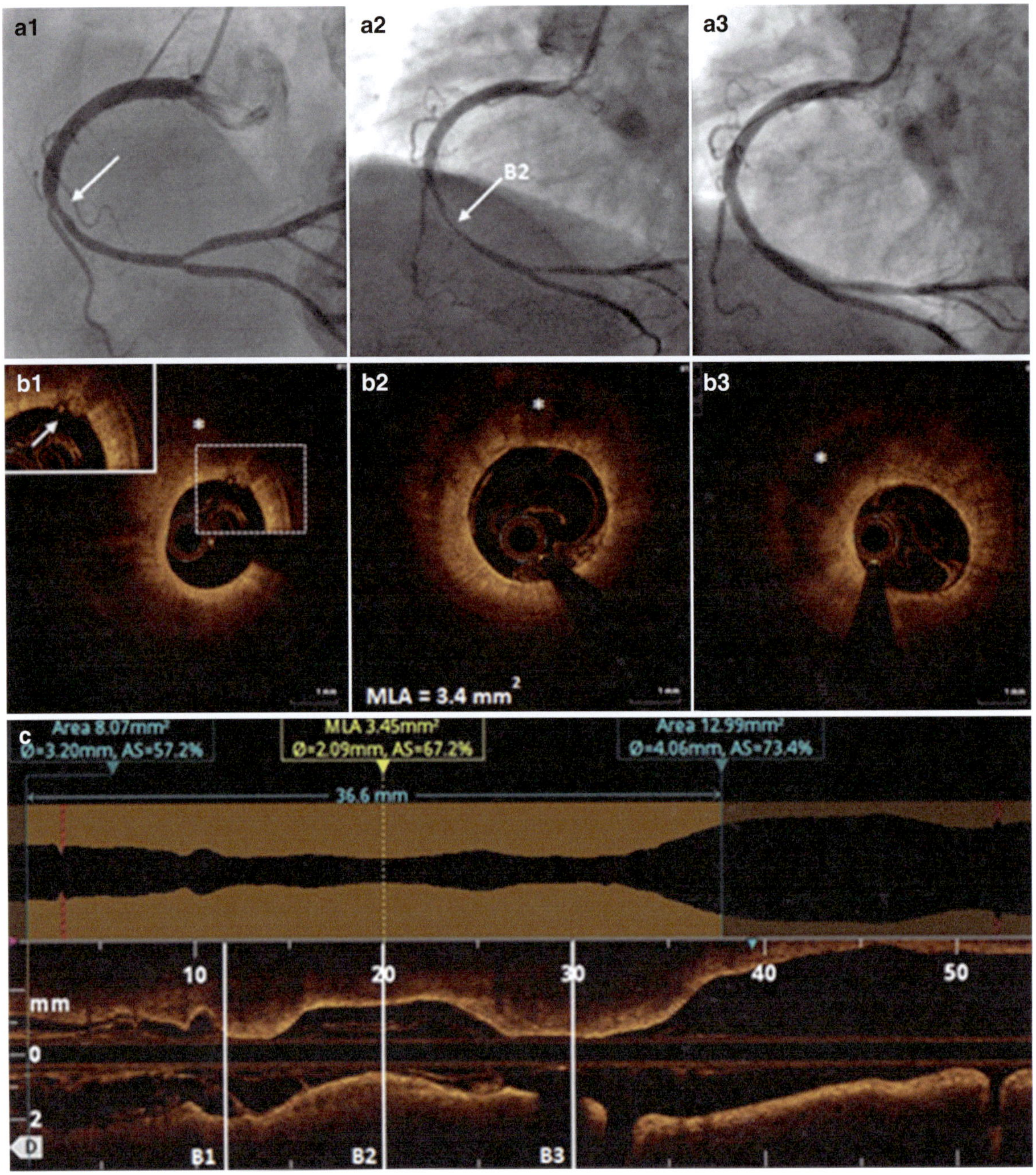

Fig. 2.19 A 66-year-old man who was an ex-smoker with controlled hypertension and hyperlipidemia and a history of chest pain presented with angina at rest. One year prior the patient was diagnosed with non-obstructive CAD with mild diffuse disease in the proximal LAD (FFR = 0.94) and distal RCA (FFR = 0.91). The previous year's angiography of the RCA is shown in a1 (*arrow*). Angiographic assessment on admission did not detect any changes in the extent of atherosclerosis in the LAD; there was, however, significant progression of the disease in the RCA with a long diffuse 70–80% stenosis in the distal portion of the vessel (**a2**, *arrow*). OCT pullback of the segment identified a 20-mm intramural hematoma (**b1**–**b3**, *asterisk*). Although no second lumen was visualized by OCT, a possible site of intimal tear was identified distally (**b1**, *inset arrow*). The minimal lumen area was 3.4 mm^2. Based on OCT assessment of lesion morphology and quantitative measurements for lesion length and reference diameters (**c**), a 4/33 mm DES was implanted in the vessel with good angiographic result (**a3**). In this case, angiography was not able to uncover the etiology of the unstable angina. By detecting a small intimal dissection and an intramural hematoma, OCT identified SCAD as a possible underlying mechanism of ACS and led to stent implantation as a preferred treatment

References

1. Virmani R, Kolodgie FD, Burke AP, Farb A, Schwartz SM. Lessons from sudden coronary death: a comprehensive morphological classification scheme for atherosclerotic lesions. Arterioscler Thromb Vasc Biol. 2000;20:1262–75.
2. Virmani R, Burke AP, Farb A, Kolodgie FD. Pathology of the vulnerable plaque. J Am Coll Cardiol. 2006;47:C13–8.
3. van der Wal AC, Becker AE, van der Loos CM, Das PK. Site of intimal rupture or erosion of thrombosed coronary atherosclerotic plaques is characterized by an inflammatory process irrespective of the dominant plaque morphology. Circulation. 1994;89:36–44.
4. Kramer MC, Rittersma SZ, de Winter RJ, Ladich ER, Fowler DR, Liang YH, et al. Relationship of thrombus healing to underlying plaque morphology in sudden coronary death. J Am Coll Cardiol. 2010;55:122–32.
5. Yonetsu T, Kakuta T, Lee T, Takahashi K, Kawaguchi N, Yamamoto G, et al. In vivo critical fibrous cap thickness for rupture-prone coronary plaques assessed by optical coherence tomography. Eur Heart J. 2011;32:1251–9.
6. Tanaka A, Imanishi T, Kitabata H, Takahashi K, Kawaguchi N, Yamamoto G, et al. Morphology of exertion-triggered plaque rupture in patients with acute coronary syndrome: an optical coherence tomography study. Circulation. 2008;118:2368–73.
7. Jia H, Abtahian F, Aguirre AD, Lee S, Chia S, Lowe H, et al. In vivo diagnosis of plaque erosion and calcified nodule in patients with acute coronary syndrome by intravascular optical coherence tomography. J Am Coll Cardiol. 2013;62:1748–58.
8. Saia F, Komukai K, Capodanno D, Sirbu V, Musumeci G, Boccuzzi G, et al. Eroded versus ruptured plaques at the culprit site of STEMI: in vivo pathophysiological features and response to primary PCI. JACC Cardiovasc Imaging. 2015;8:566–75.
9. Higuma T, Soeda T, Abe N, Yamada M, Yokoyama H, Shibutani S, et al. A combined optical coherence tomography and intravascular ultrasound study on plaque rupture, plaque erosion, and calcified nodule in patients with ST-segment elevation myocardial infarction: incidence, morphologic characteristics, and outcomes after percutaneous coronary intervention. JACC Cardiovasc Interv. 2015;8:1166–76.
10. Ozaki Y, Okumura M, Ismail TF, Motoyama S, Naruse H, Hattori K, et al. Coronary CT angiographic characteristics of culprit lesions in acute coronary syndromes not related to plaque rupture as defined by optical coherence tomography and angioscopy. Eur Heart J. 2011;32:2814–23.
11. Otsuka F, Joner M, Prati F, Virmani R, Narula J. Clinical classification of plaque morphology in coronary disease. Nat Rev Cardiol. 2014;11:379–89.
12. Kanwar SS, Stone GW, Singh M, Virmani R, Olin J, Akasaka T, et al. Acute coronary syndromes without coronary plaque rupture. Nat Rev Cardiol. 2016;13:257–65.
13. Prati F, Uemura S, Souteyrand G, Virmani R, Motreff P, Di Vito L, et al. OCT-based diagnosis and management of STEMI associated with intact fibrous cap. JACC Cardiovasc Imaging. 2013;6:283–7.
14. Holmes DR Jr, Lerman A, Moreno PR, King SB 3rd, Sharma SK. Diagnosis and management of STEMI arising from plaque erosion. JACC Cardiovasc Imaging. 2013;6:290–6.
15. Braunwald E. Coronary plaque erosion: recognition and management. JACC Cardiovasc Imaging. 2013;6:288–9.
16. Kamran M, Guptan A, Bogal M. Spontaneous coronary artery dissection: case series and review. J Invasive Cardiol. 2008;20:553–9.
17. Aqel RA, Zoghbi GJ, Iskandrian A. Spontaneous coronary artery dissection, aneurysms, and pseudoaneurysms: a review. Echocardiography. 2004;21:175–82.
18. Jorgensen MB, Aharonian V, Mansukhani P, Mahrer PR. Spontaneous coronary dissection: a cluster of cases with this rare finding. Am Heart J. 1994;127:1382–7.
19. Manalo-Estrella P, Barker AE. Histopathologic findings in human aortic media associated with pregnancy. Arch Pathol. 1967;83:336–41.
20. Alfonso F, Paulo M, Gonzalo N, Dutary J, Jimenez-Quevedo P, Lennie V, et al. Diagnosis of spontaneous coronary artery dissection by optical coherence tomography. J Am Coll Cardiol. 2012;59:1073–9.
21. Roleder T, Sharma R, Kini AS, Moreno P, Sharma SK. Imaging of postpartum coronary artery's spontaneous dissection treated with stents implantation. Eur Heart J Cardiovasc Imaging. 2013;14:503.
22. Egred M, Viswanathan G, Davis GK. Myocardial infarction in young adults. Postgrad Med J. 2005;81:741–5.
23. Sinicato NA, da Silva Cardoso PA, Appenzeller S. Risk factors in cardiovascular disease in systemic lupus erythematosus. Curr Cardiol Rev. 2013;9:15–9.
24. Oliva PB, Potts DE, Pluss RG. Coronary arterial spasm in Prinzmetal angina. Documentation by coronary arteriography. N Engl J Med. 1973;288:745–51.
25. Roberts WC, Curry RC Jr, Isner JM, Waller BF, McManus BM, Mariani-Costantini R, Ross AM. Sudden death in Prinzmetal's angina with coronary spasm documented by angiography. Analysis of three necropsy patients. Am J Cardiol. 1982;50:203–10.
26. Lanza GA, Careri G, Crea F. Mechanisms of coronary artery spasm. Circulation. 2011;124:1774–82.
27. Figueras J, Domingo E, Ferreira I, Lidon RM, Garcia-Dorado D. Persistent angina pectoris, cardiac mortality and myocardial infarction during a 12 year follow-up in 273 variant angina patients without significant fixed coronary stenosis. Am J Cardiol. 2012;110:1249–55.
28. Kobayashi N, Takano M, Hata N, Yamamoto M, Shinada T, Takahashi Y, et al. Optical coherence tomography findings in a case of acute coronary syndrome caused by coronary vasospasm. Int Heart J. 2010;51:291–2.
29. Morikawa Y, Uemura S, Ishigami K, Soeda T, Okayama S, Takemoto Y, et al. Morphological features of coronary arteries in patients with coronary spastic angina: assessment with intracoronary optical coherence tomography. Int J Cardiol. 2011;146:334–40.
30. Kohno H, Sueda S, Sakaue T. Separation of the intima-media complex from the adventitia during spontaneous coronary artery spasm documented by intracoronary optical coherence tomography. Int J Cardiol. 2012;154:e4–5.
31. Vizzi V, Johnson TW, Jenkins N, Strange JW, Baumbach A. Dynamic separation of coronary artery medial and adventitial layers with vasospasm: new insights using OCT. Int J Cardiol. 2013;167:2344–5.
32. Yahagi K, Zarpak R, Sakakura K, Otsuka F, Kutys R, Ladich E, et al. Multiple simultaneous plaque erosion in 3 coronary arteries. JACC Cardiovasc Imaging. 2014;7:1172–4.

Stable Coronary Artery Disease: Assistance in Complex Percutaneous Coronary Intervention

3

3.1 Introduction

Optical coherence tomography (OCT) has been increasingly used in clinical practice as a guide during percutaneous coronary intervention (PCI). Prior to stent implantation, OCT can provide accurate measurements of the minimal lumen area, the distal and proximal reference areas, and lesion length. The accuracy of the OCT measurements has been established by the ex vivo lumen diameter assessment of Plexiglas phantoms [1]. The minimal lumen area (MLA) measured by OCT in vivo was slightly smaller than intravascular ultrasound (IVUS)-MLA, but the correlation between the two measurements was highly significant ($r = 0.82$; $p < 0.001$) [2]. OCT showed excellent reproducibility for both the lumen area and the lesion length measurements with low intraobserver, interobserver, and interpullback variability [3, 4]. Fully automatic computer-assisted lumen contour detection in OCT images has been shown to represent a reliable tool for in vivo assessment of stented coronary vessels [5, 6]. These preprocedural measurements can help select stent and balloon sizes.

OCT is particularly useful during challenging procedures, such as calcified lesions, bifurcation, and unprotected left main (ULM) PCI. OCT imaging can help characterize lesion morphology and select treatment strategy based on plaque characteristics. It is being proposed that lipid-rich lesions may be amenable to medical therapy and resolution of luminal obstruction verified by improved fractional flow reserve (FFR) [7]. PCI of calcified lesions has been associated with lower rates of procedural success and higher rates of subsequent adverse cardiovascular events [8]. Because of reduction in vessel wall compliance, calcified lesions have higher risks of stent underexpansion and malapposition and acute postprocedural complications such as dissection and perforation. Development of atheroablation techniques, in particular rotational and orbital atherectomy, significantly improved the success rate of calcified lesion PCI. OCT allows measurements of calcification size and depth and their precise location within the lesion, which might help select the appropriate atheroablation technique.

Treatment of coronary artery bifurcation lesions remains a challenging area in interventional cardiology despite major advances in bifurcation stenting approach [9, 10]. Side branch (SB) occlusion can result in vessel closure and ischemia, leading to increased incidence of periprocedural myocardial infarction (MI) and even cardiac deaths after PCI [11]. Provisional stenting remains the main approach to treatment of bifurcation lesions; however, it may result in significant narrowing of the SB ostium after main vessel stenting. High-resolution OCT imaging can characterize SB stenosis before and after stenting, select appropriate treatment strategy, and evaluate the effects of SB treatment. Three-dimensional OCT reconstruction provides a unique opportunity to assess the true morphology of the main and side vessels [12]. Preprocedure assessment of bifurcation lesion morphology with OCT can help identify SBs with a high risk of occlusion. The presence of large lipid plaque in the proximal segment of the main vessel (MV) has been shown to be an independent OCT predictor of SB stenosis severity after MV stenting [13, 14].

Coronary artery bypass graft (CABG) surgery has historically been the treatment of choice for patients with unprotected left main coronary artery (LMCA) disease. However, with the introduction of drug-eluting stents (DESs), selected patients with unprotected LMCAs have been increasingly treated with PCI [15, 16]. A recent pilot trial demonstrated the safety and feasibility of frequency-domain OCT for unprotected left main PCI [17]. Compared to IVUS, OCT provided a similar assessment of lumen and stent dimensions

Electronic Supplementary Material The online version of this chapter (doi:10.1007/978-3-319-62666-6_3) contains supplementary material, which is available to authorized users.

A. Kini et al., *Atlas of Coronary Intravascular Optical Coherence Tomography*, DOI 10.1007/978-3-319-62666-6_3

but was more sensitive in detecting malapposition and edge dissections.

Finally, OCT imaging before stenting can provide patient risk stratification for periprocedural MI, since OCT-derived thin-cap fibroatheroma and evidence of plaque rupture have been associated with elevation of post-PCI myocardial necrosis markers [18, 19]. Compared to plaque burden by intravascular ultrasound (IVUS) and plaque lipid content by near infrared spectroscopy (NIRS), OCT fibrous cap thickness was the most important independent predictor of periprocedural MI in a recent multimodality imaging study [20].

3.2 Case 1. Rotational Atherectomy of a Proximal LAD Lesion: Grinding the Lesion (Figs. 3.1 and 3.2, Videos 3.1 (Part I), 3.1 (Part II), 3.2, and 3.3)

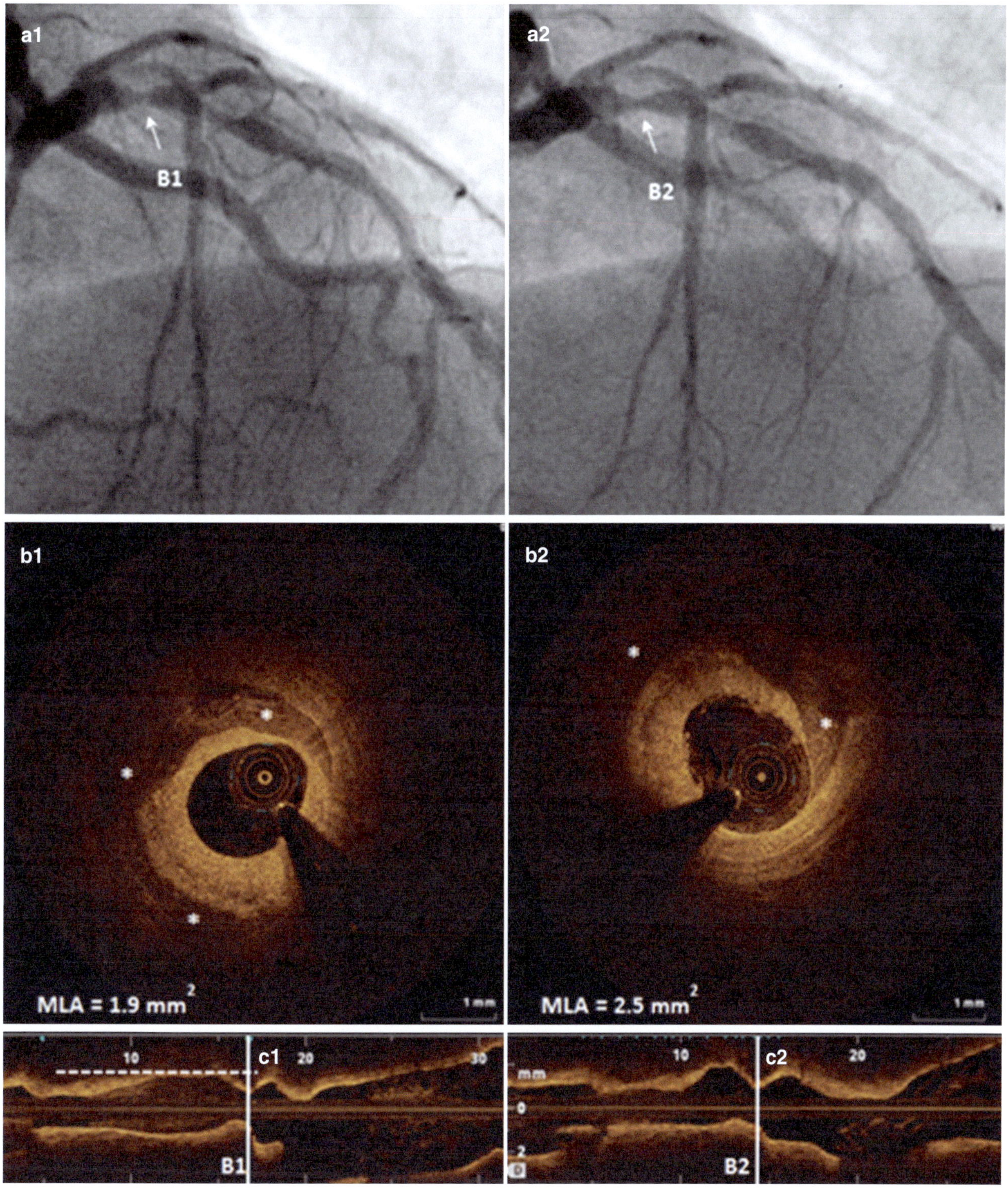

Fig. 3.1 A 47-year-old male, a smoker with hyperlipidemia and hypertension with a positive single-photon emission computed tomography myocardial perfusion imaging (SPECT-MPI) and LAD stenosis on coronary computed tomography angiography (CTA) and was found to have stable angina. The coronary angiogram showed a 70–80% stenosis of the proximal LAD with calcification (**a1**, *arrow*). OCT imaging confirmed the presence of severe calcification at the site of stenosis with a minimal lumen area of 1.9 mm^2 (**b1**, *asterisk*) and proximal to the MLA with a total length of 14 mm (**c1**, *dotted line*). Calcified plaque was ablated by rotational atherectomy (RA) using a 1.75-mm burr for 60 s. OCT pullback performed after RA demonstrated a 32% increase in the minimal lumen area (**b1** vs. **b2**), uniform plaque modification with a smooth cylindrical shape of the lumen (**c2**), and small intimal cuts (**b2**)

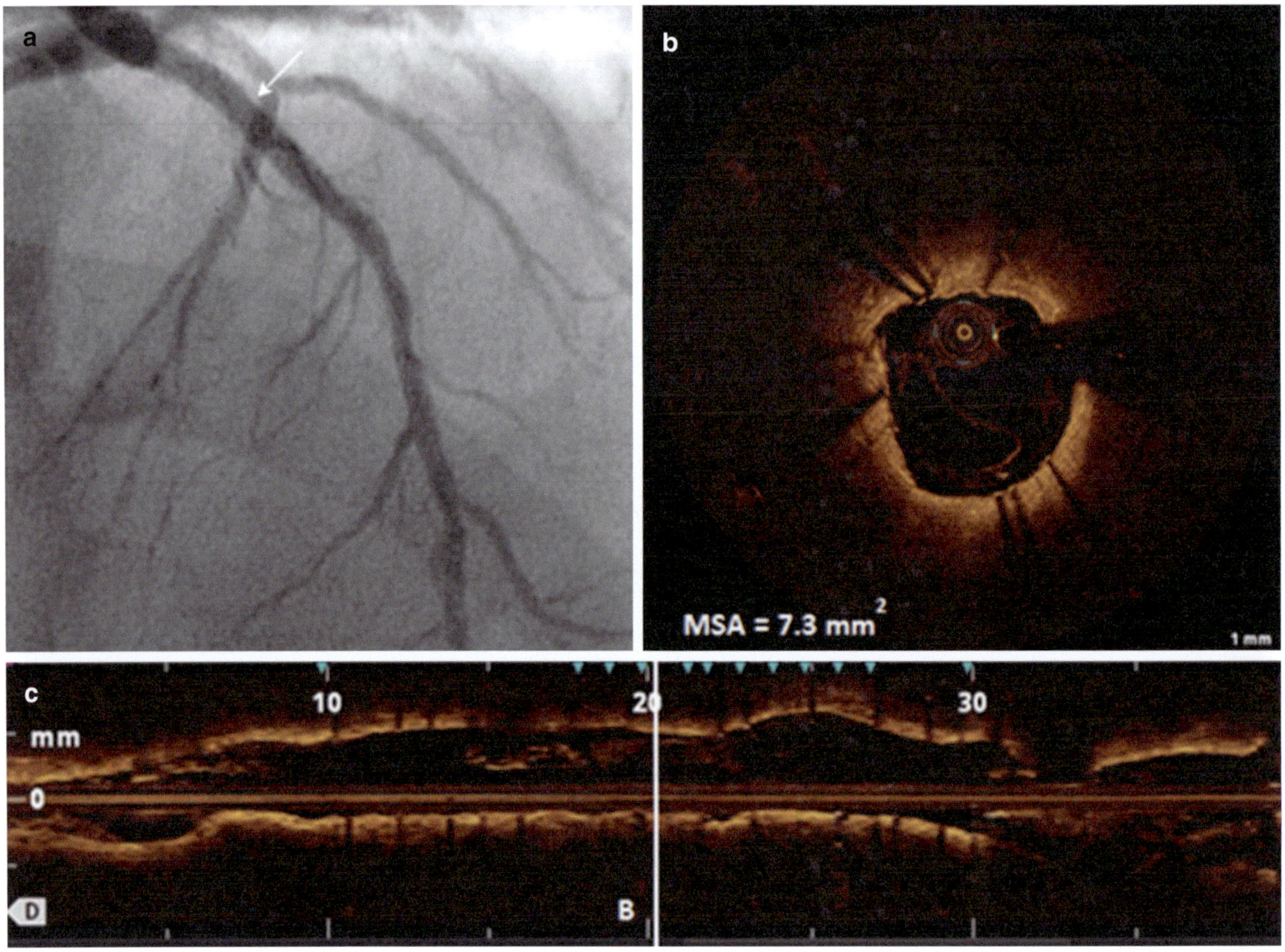

Fig. 3.2 Coronary angiogram and OCT after stenting. An everolimus-eluting stent (3.5/24 mm) was implanted with a successful result on angiography (**a**). Postintervention OCT imaging confirmed good stent apposition and expansion with minimal stent area (MSA) of 7.3 mm^2 (**b**, **c**)

3.3 Case 2. Orbital Atherectomy of a Heavily Calcified RCA Lesion: Shaving the Lesion (Figs. 3.3 and 3.4, Videos 3.4, 3.5, and 3.6)

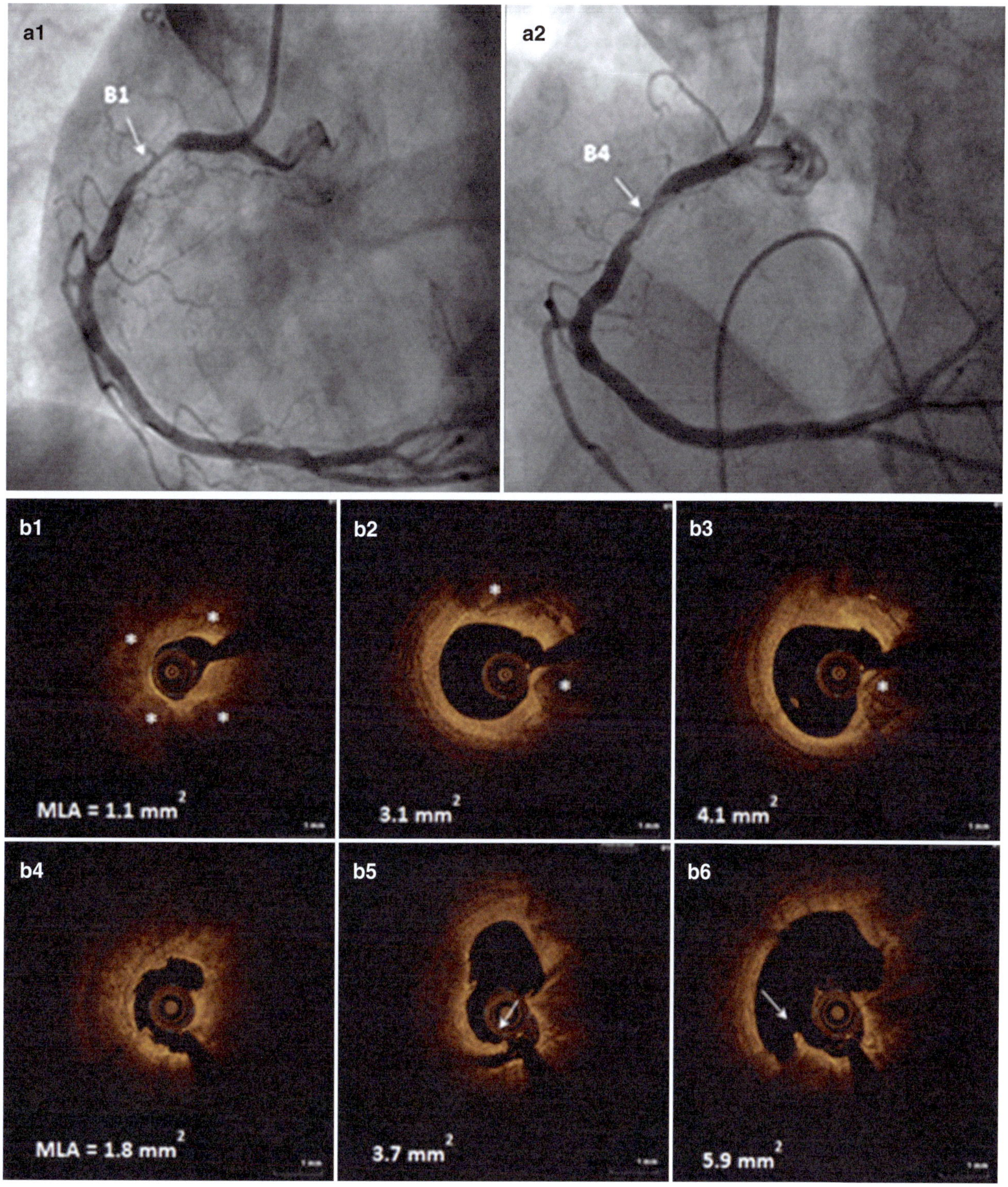

Fig. 3.3 A 64-year-old male who was a smoker with hyperlipidemia and hypertension and recent NSTEMI PCI to the proximal LAD presented with persistent chest pain. Abnormal stress MPI showed mild to moderate inferior ischemia. A coronary angiogram demonstrated a 70–80% occlusion of the proximal RCA with severe calcification (**a1**, *arrow*). Pre-PCI OCT imaging revealed circumferential calcification at the site of minimal lumen area (**b1**, *asterisks*) and moderate calcification proximal to the MLA (**b2**, **b3**, *asterisks*). Orbital atherectomy (OA) was performed with a 1.25-mm classic crown at 80,000 rpm for 40 s followed by 120,000 rpm for 40 s, resulting in acute lumen gain by angiography (**a2**, *arrow*). OCT imaging after atherectomy confirmed effective calcium debulking with a 64% increase in minimal lumen area (**b1** vs. **b4**) and significant modifications of fibrocalcific plaques (**b5**, **b6**, *arrow*)

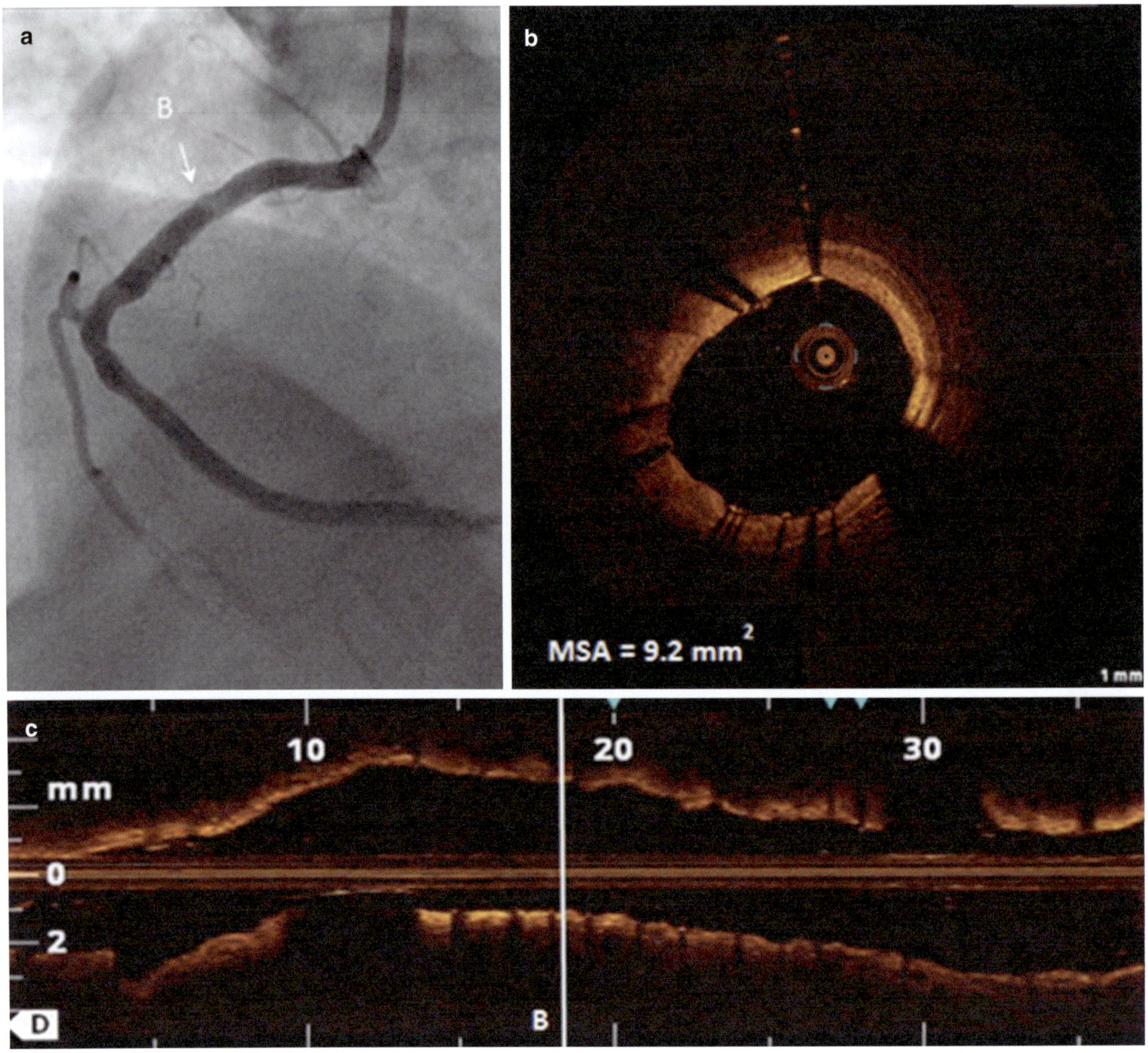

Fig. 3.4 Final post-PCI angiogram and OCT pullback were performed after a 4/23 mm everolimus eluting stent was implanted in the proximal RCA with a successful result by angiography (**a**) and OCT imaging (**b**, **c**)

3.4 Case 3. Orbital Atherectomy for Proximal LAD In-Stent Restenosis: Debulking an Iatrogenic Complication (Figs. 3.5 and 3.6, Videos 3.7 and 3.8)

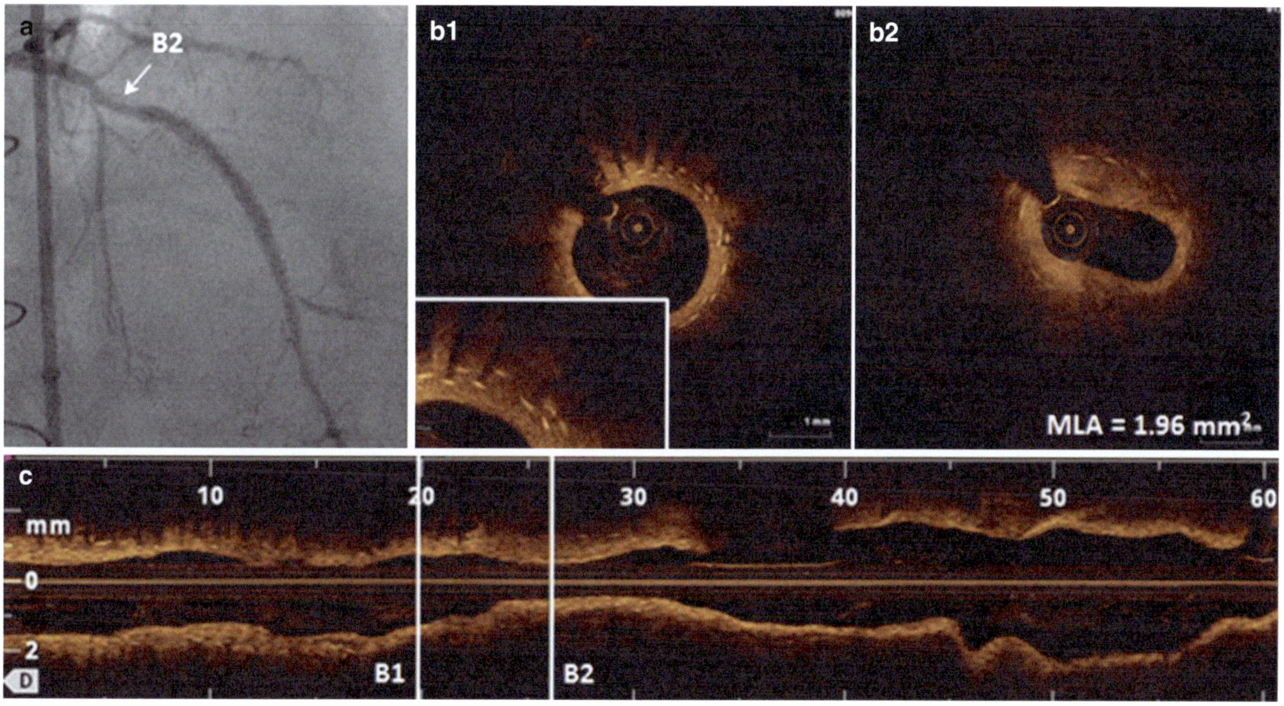

Fig. 3.5 A 67-year-old female with hyperlipidemia, controlled hypertension, and insulin-dependent diabetes mellitus (IDDM) was admitted with crescendo angina on maximal medical therapy and abnormal SPECT MPI demonstrating ischemia involving the anterior wall. The patient had a prior history of MI, CABG, and multiple PCIs. The last PCI of the mid LAD with a 3/38 mm DES was performed 6 months prior to the procedure. Coronary angiography revealed a significant in-stent restenosis lesion in the proximal LAD (**a**, *arrow*). An in-stent restenosis lesion with mostly homogeneous neointima was revealed by OCT; the minimal lumen area of the lesion was 1.96 mm^2 (**b2**, **c**). A smaller amount of neointima and two stent layers were visualized by OCT in the segment distal to the MLA site (**b1**, *inset*)

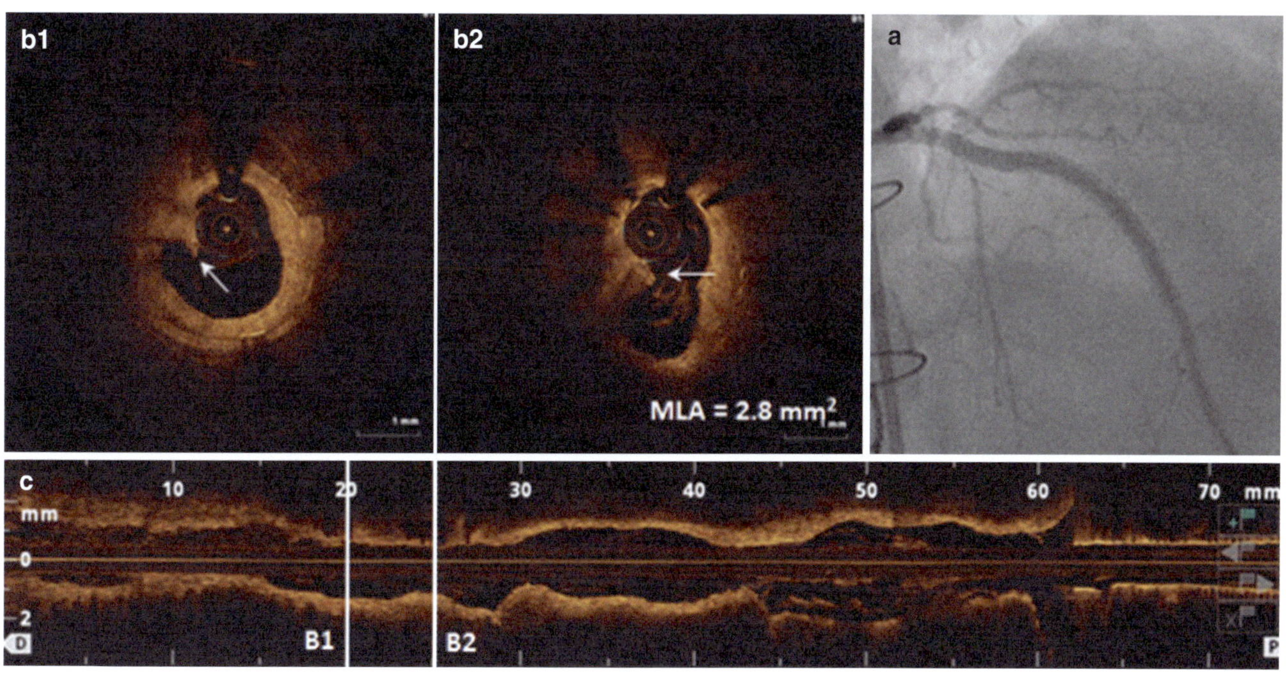

Fig. 3.6 Postatherectomy OCT images and final poststenting angiogram. The lesion was treated with orbital atherectomy (OA) using a 1.25-mm classic crown at 80,000 rpm for 105 s followed by a cutting balloon (CB). Post-treatment OCT images demonstrated effective plaque removal (**b1**, **b2**, **c**, *arrow*) leading to acute lumen gain characterized by a 43% increase in the minimal lumen area (**b2**). A 3.5/18 mm everolimus eluting stent was deployed in the proximal LAD with a satisfactory angiographic result (**a**)

3.5 Case 4. Single Stenting of LAD-D1 Bifurcation Followed by Simultaneous Two-Balloon Inflation: About Kissing to Perfection (Figs. 3.7 and 3.8, Videos 3.9 and 3.10)

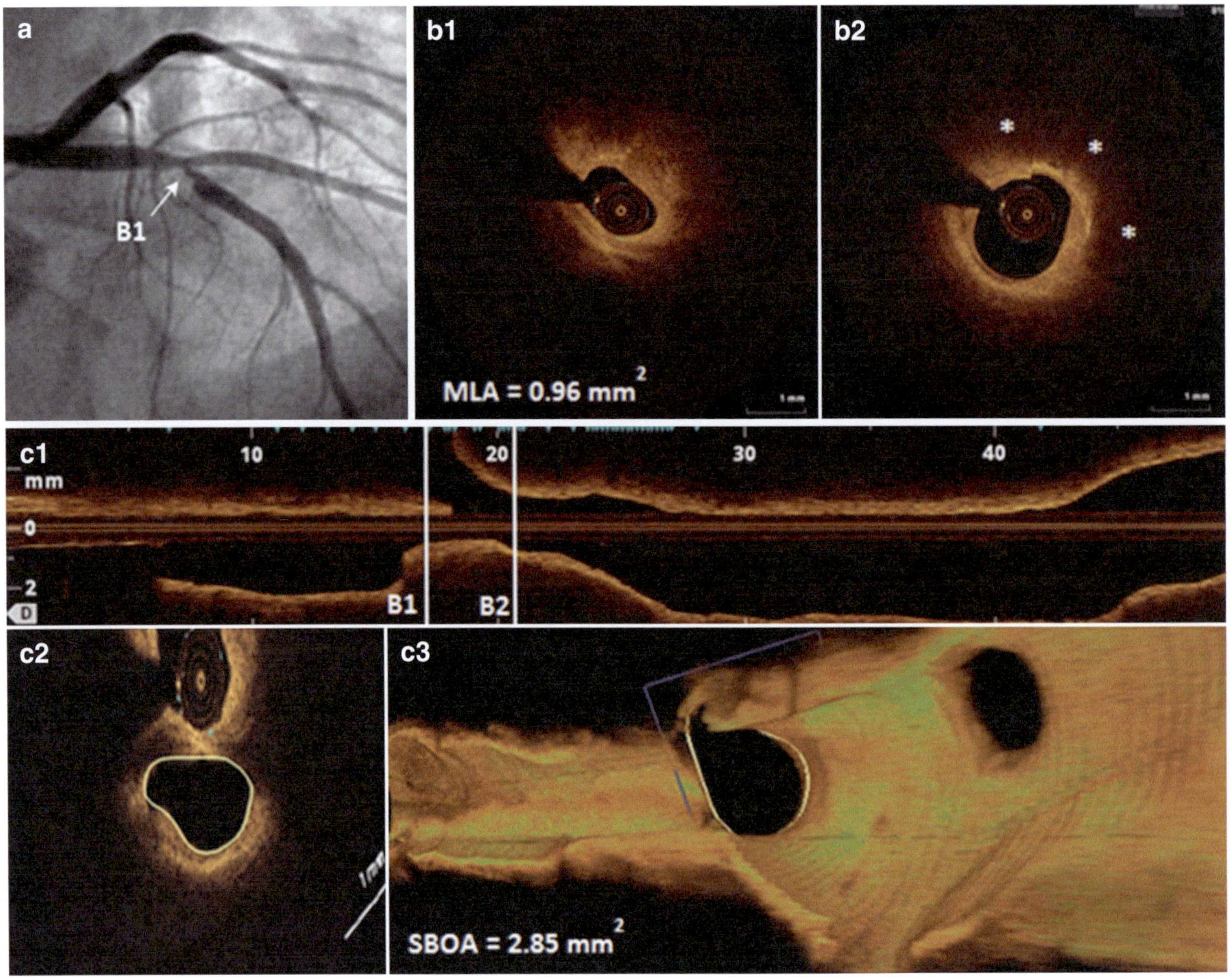

Fig. 3.7 Coronary angiography, two- and three-dimensional OCT images before stenting. An 83-year-old male presented with exercise-induced chest discomfort. The patient's medical history included controlled hypertension. Computed tomography angiography (CTA) showed severe LAD stenosis and SPECT MPI detected inducible myocardial ischemia. Coronary angiography demonstrated a mid LAD bifurcation lesion, Medina classification (1.1.1) (**a**, *arrow*). A large lipid-rich plaque proximal to the bifurcation area was detected by OCT (**b2**, *asterisks*). Mostly fibrotic plaque was visualized at the site of the MLA = 0.96 mm^2 (**b1**). Since only mild calcification was detected by OCT, no atherectomy was performed. The side branch ostium area (SBOA) was 2.85 mm^2 before PCI by three-dimensional OCT cut plane analysis (**c2**, **c3**, *circled*)

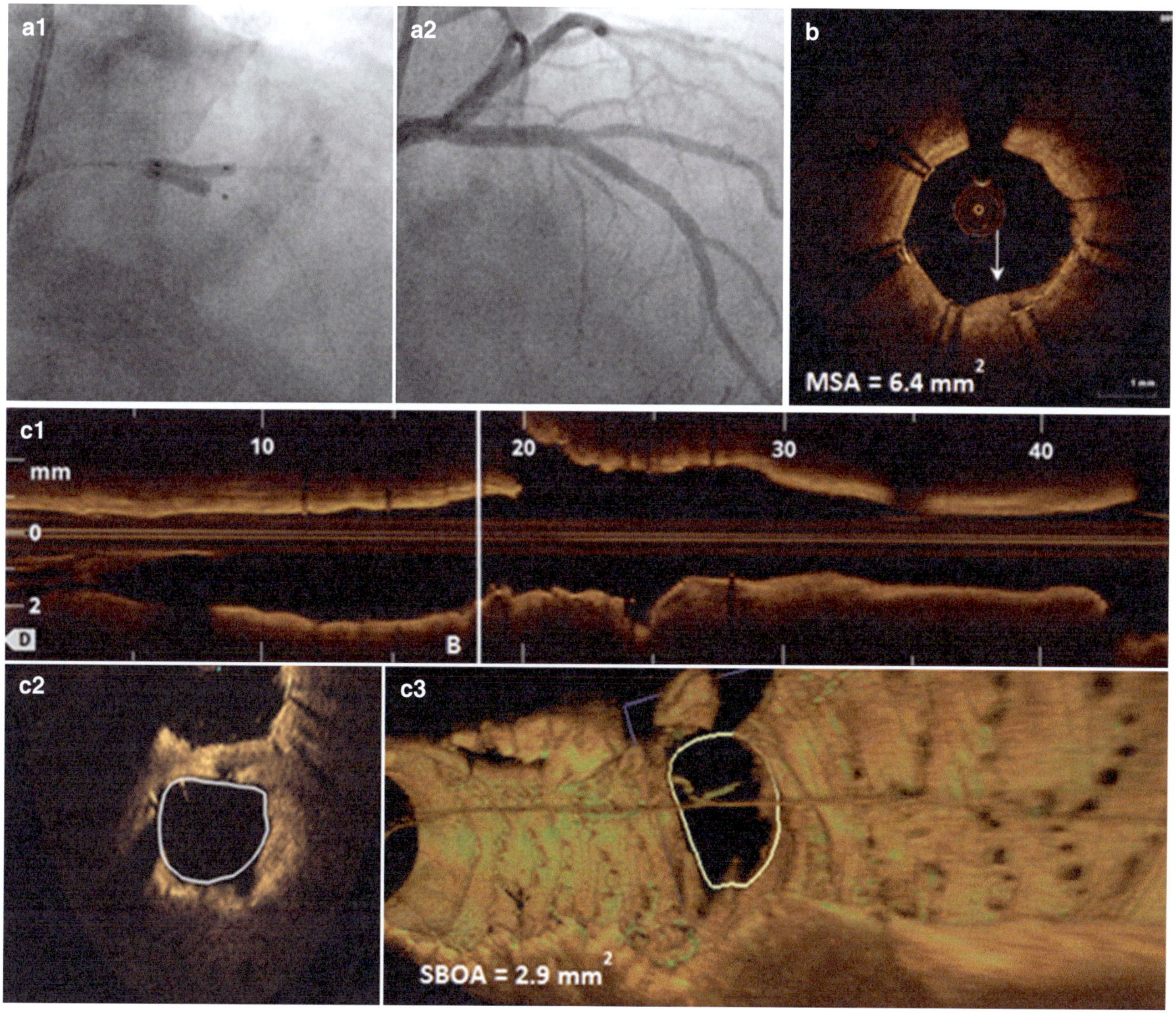

Fig. 3.8 Coronary angiogram, two-dimensional and three-dimensional OCT images after stenting. This bifurcation region was treated by single stenting with kissing balloon inflation (**a1**). The postprocedural coronary angiogram showed no dissection in the side branch (**a2**). OCT pullback of the main vessel showed good stent apposition and expansion with a minimal stent area of 6.4 mm^2 (**b**, *arrow*). There was no change in the side branch ostium area after PCI as assessed by three-dimensional OCT (**c2**, **c3** *circled*)

3.6 Case 5. Compromised Side Branch Flow After LAD-D1 Stenting: On Finding Faults and Correcting Consequences (Figs. 3.9, 3.10, and 3.11, Videos 3.11, 3.12, and 3.13)

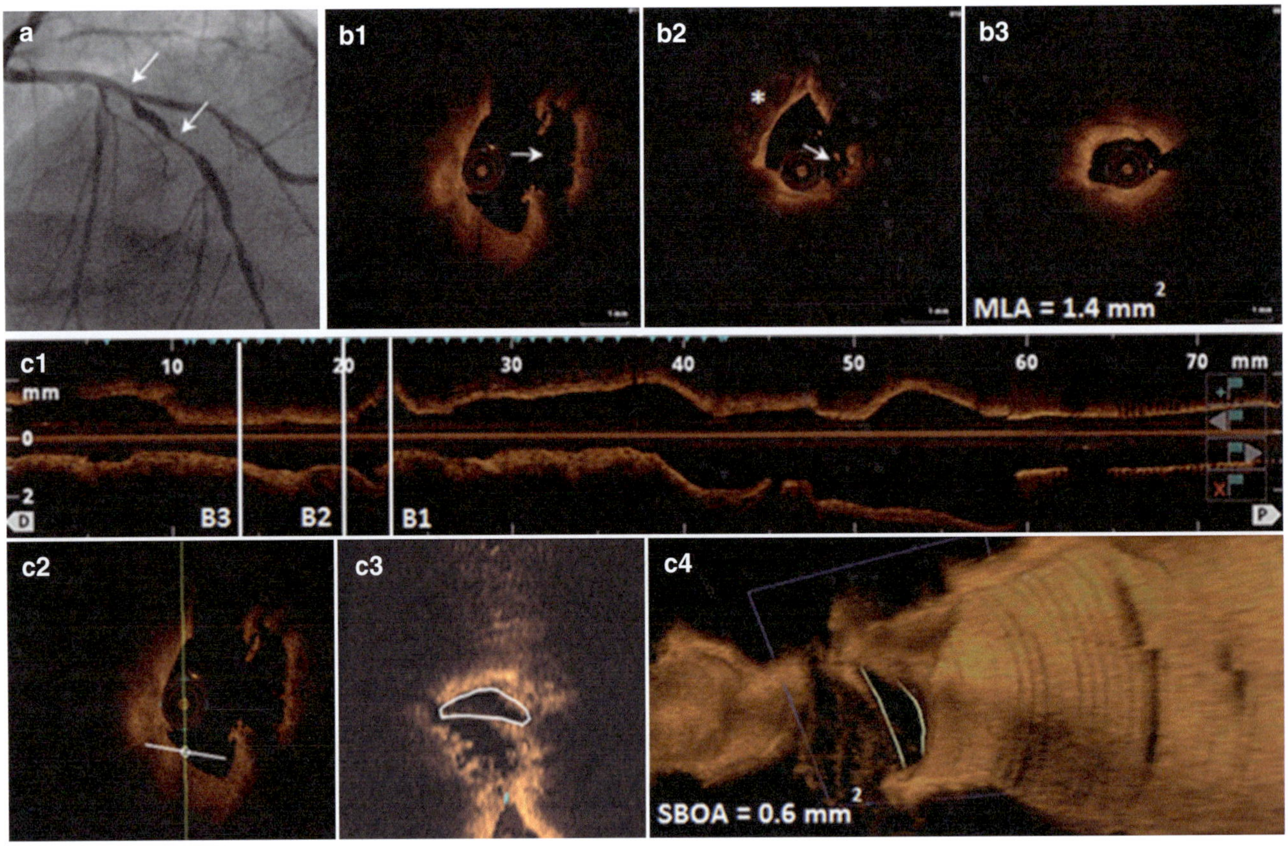

Fig. 3.9 Coronary angiography and OCT imaging before stenting. A 66-year-old male with a history of controlled hypertension, hyperlipidemia, and smoking presented with CCS class II angina on optimal medical therapy and three-vessel disease on coronary CTA. Coronary angiography demonstrated a 70–80% stenosis and severe calcification in the proximal and mid LAD (**a**, *arrows*). Rotational atherectomy (RA) was performed with a 1.5-mm burr in the proximal and a 1.25-mm burr in the mid LAD. OCT pullback after RA visualized a fibrocalcific lesion with an MLA of 1.4 mm^2 (**b3**) and moderate to severe calcification (**b2**, *asterisk*). Significant post-RA tissue modifications were visualized in the bifurcation area (**b1**, **b2**, *arrow*). Side branch ostium area (SBOA) after RA before stenting was 0.6 mm^2 by three-dimensional OCT cut-plane analysis (**c2**-**c4**, *circled*)

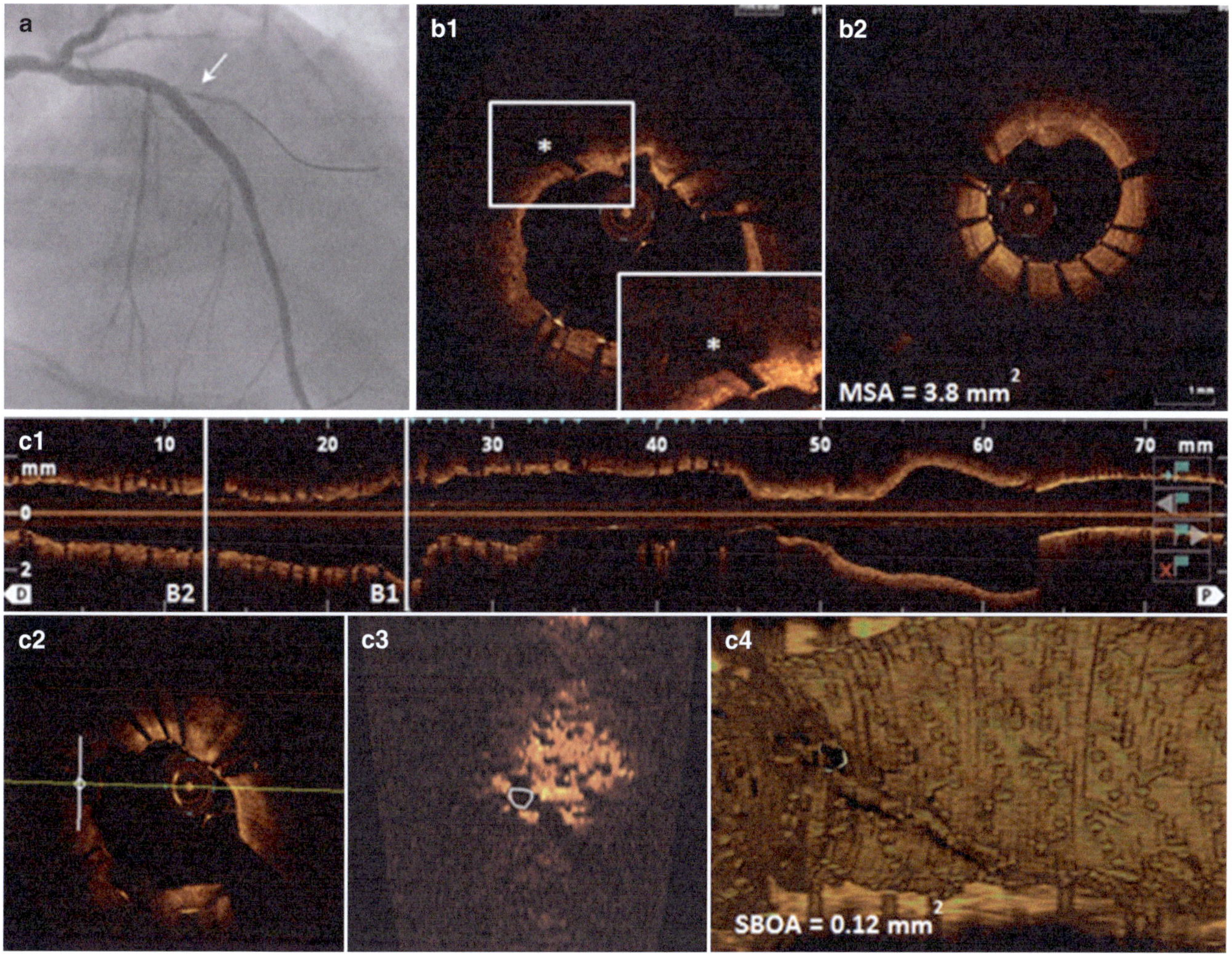

Fig. 3.10 Coronary angiography, two- and three-dimensional OCT imaging after stenting. The main vessel lesions were treated with two drug-eluting stents (3/28 and 2.75/38 mm), which resulted in thrombolysis in myocardial Infarction (TIMI) 2 flow in the first diagonal branch (**a**, *arrow*). OCT imaging of the main vessel after stenting visualized a jailed side branch (**b1**, *inset, asterisk*). Three-dimensional OCT reconstruction of the stented segment revealed significant reduction of SB ostium from 0.6 mm^2 before stenting to 0.12 mm^2 after intervention (**c2**-**c4**, *circled*). Since there was no evidence for the side branch ostial dissection or spasm, the mechanism of SB occlusion was classified as coronary plaque and/or carina shift, and the operator proceeded with kissing balloon postdilatation to restore the SB flow

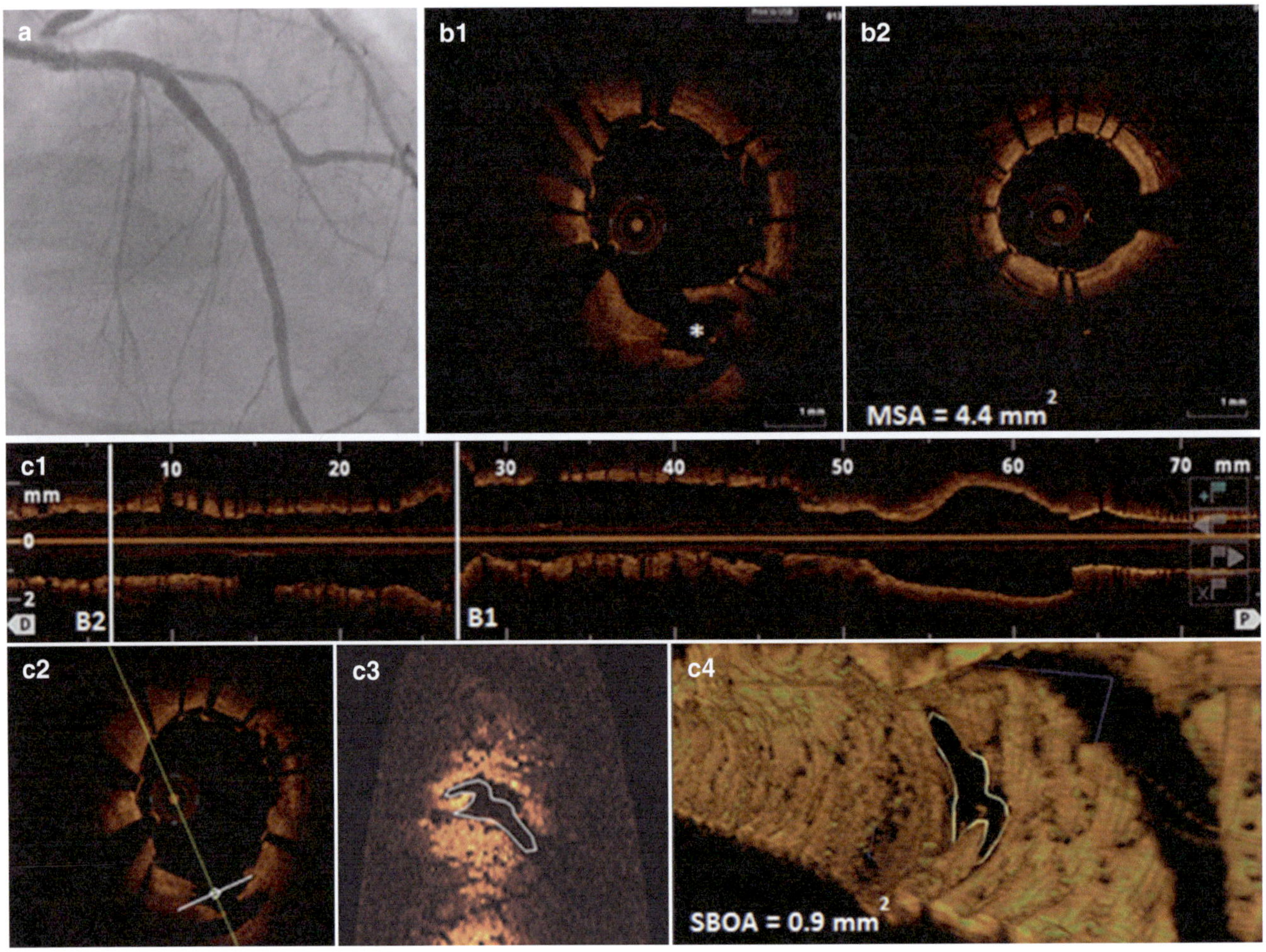

Fig. 3.11 Coronary angiography and OCT imaging after kissing balloon inflation (KBI). KBI of mid LAD and D1 was performed with 2.75/20 and 2/15 mm balloons. As a result, TIMI 3 flow was restored in the SB (**a**) and SB ostium area was increased from 0.12 to 0.9 mm^2 (**b1**, *asterisk;* **c3**-**c4**, *circled*). In addition, there was an improved stent expansion with MSA increased from 3.8 to 4.4 mm^2 (**b2**). In this case, OCT imaging helped identify the mechanism responsibly for SB occlusion as plaque/carina shift, which led to KBI as the preferred treatment to restore the flow. Three-dimensional OCT reconstruction of the bifurcation lesion allowed assessment of the effect of treatment on the SB ostium area

3.7 Case 6. V Stenting of LAD-D1 Bifurcation Lesion: About Metallizing the Carina (Figs. 3.12 and 3.13, Videos 3.14 and 3.15)

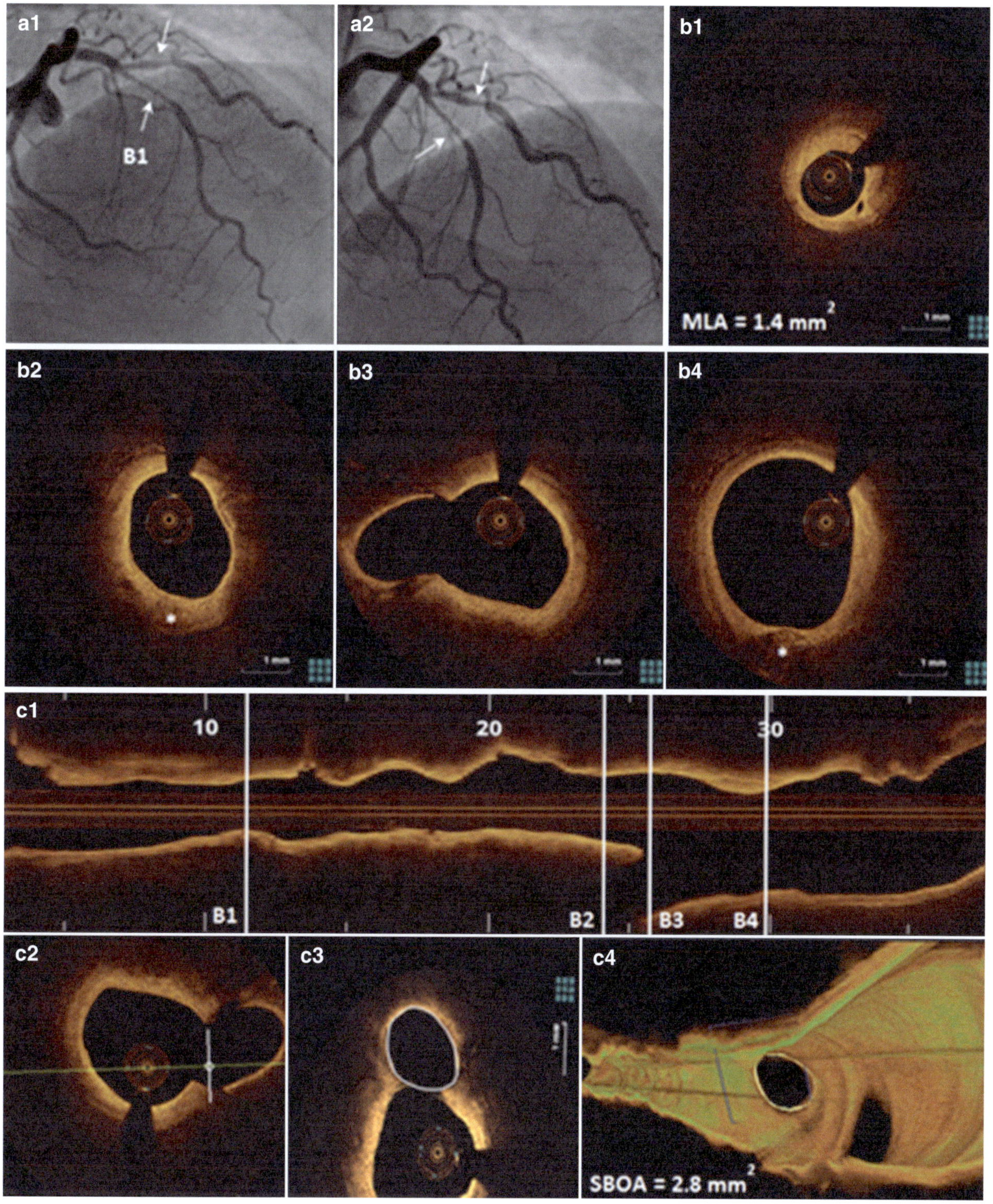

Fig. 3.12 Coronary angiography and OCT imaging before PCI. A 66-year-old female with history of controlled hypertension and dyslipidemia presented with progressive chest pain and shortness of breath on exertion for several months. SPECT MPI showed mild reversible defect of the inferoapical and inferolateral walls. Coronary angiography demonstrated a mid LAD bifurcation lesion, Medina classification (0.1.1) (**a1**, **a2**, *arrows*). OCT imaging of the main vessel demonstrated a fibrocalcific plaque with MLA of 1.4 mm^2 (**b1**) distal to the LAD-D1 bifurcation area (**b3**). There were several small calcific deposits (**b2**, **b4**, *asterisks*) detected in the vicinity of the bifurcation. Pre-PCI side branch ostium area (SBOA) was 2.8 mm^2 as measured by three-dimensional OCT cut-plane analysis (**c2–c4**, *circled*)

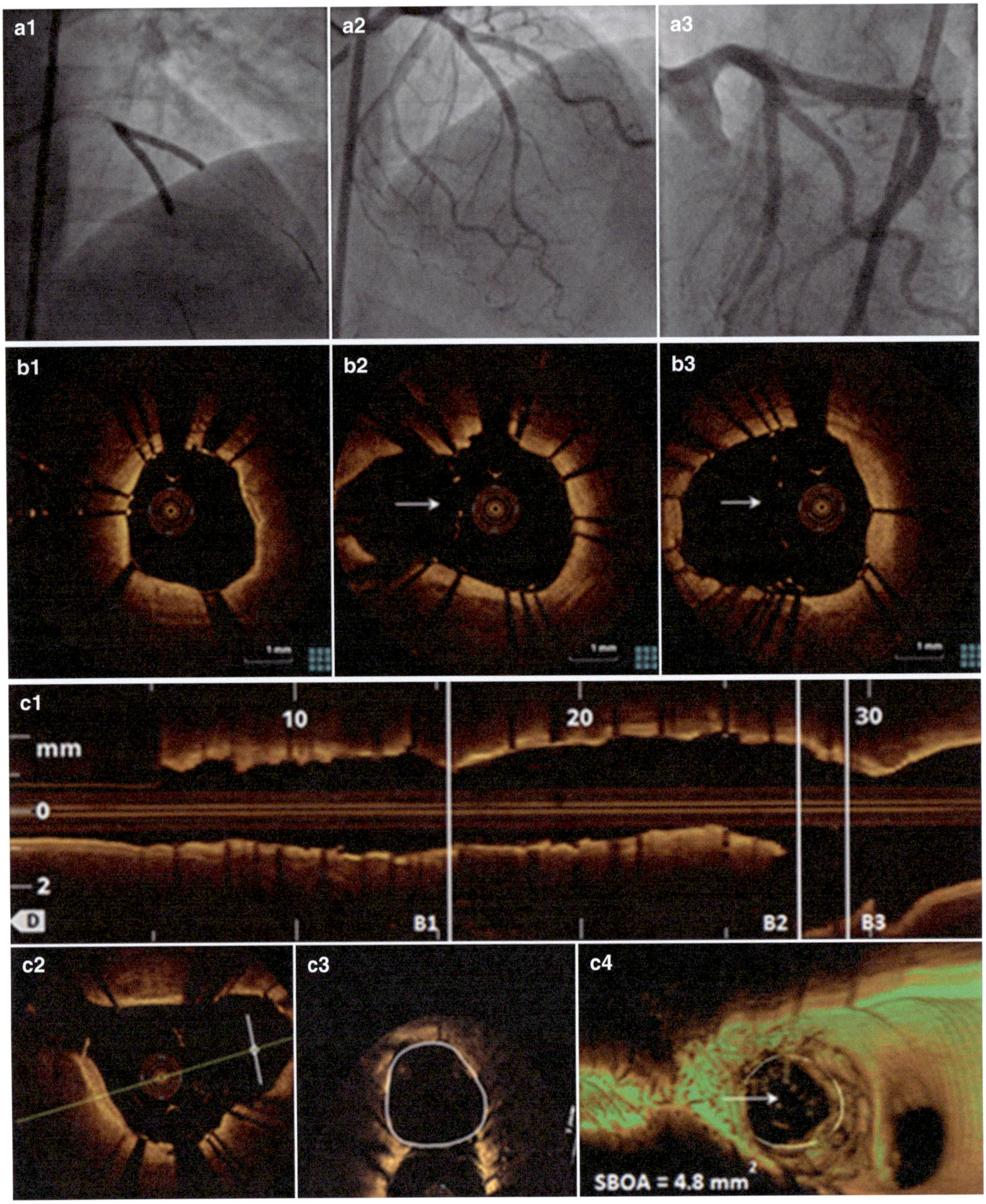

Fig. 3.13 Coronary angiography and OCT imaging after stenting. The bifurcation lesion was treated by the V stenting technique with 2.75/28 and 2.75/23 mm everolimus eluting stents for mid LAD and D1, respectively. Both stents were deployed simultaneously at 12 atm (**a1**). Postprocedural coronary angiogram showed an optimal result (**a2**, **a3**). OCT imaging of the main vessel confirmed good stent apposition and expansion with an MSA of 4.7 mm^2 without dissection at the stent edges (**b1**). In the proximal bifurcation segment, where two stents touch each other, OCT visualized a metal carina formed by floating struts (**b2**, **b3**, *white arrow*). Three-dimensional OCT cut-plane analysis showed a significant increase in SBOA after V stenting (**c3**, **c4**, *circled*) and visualized floating struts proximal to bifurcation (**c4**, *arrow*). In this case, OCT imaging before stenting helped characterize the morphology and distribution of coronary plaque around the bifurcation area to select an appropriate lesion preparation and stenting strategy, while poststenting OCT allowed assessment of the immediate effects of the intervention

3.8 Case 7. Atherectomy and Two-Stent Technique for Calcified LAD-D1 Bifurcation Lesion: Dealing Wisely with Double Whammy (Figs. 3.14 and 3.15, Videos 3.16 and 3.17)

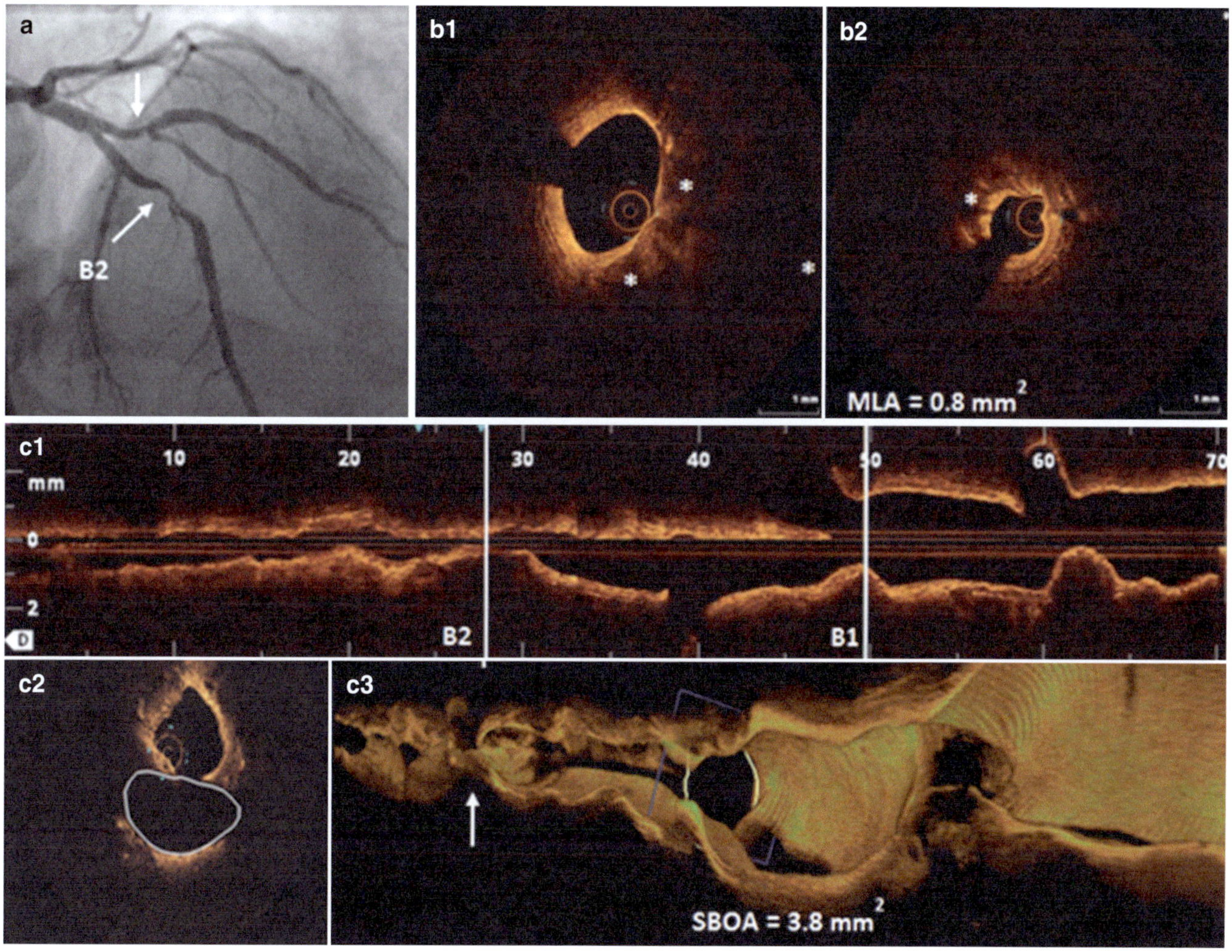

Fig. 3.14 Coronary angiography and OCT images before stenting. A 70-year-old female who was an ex-smoker with hyperlipidemia and hypothyroidism presented for a staged intervention of the LAD. Coronary angiography revealed a 95% mid LAD and 80% first diagonal calcific bifurcation lesion (**a**, *arrows*). The fractional flow reserve (FFR) values for the LAD and D1 were 0.77 and 0.78, respectively. OCT pullback of the LAD showed moderate to severe calcification around the minimal lumen area site (**b2**, *asterisk*) and bifurcation segment (**b1**, *asterisks*). The side branch ostium area (SBOA) before treatment was 3.8 mm^2 as assessed by three-dimensional OCT (**c2**, **c3**, *circled*). The *arrow* in **c3** indicates the MLA site in the three-dimensional OCT reconstruction of the segment. Based on OCT plaque characterization, the operator proceeded with rotational atherectomy followed by two-stenting strategy

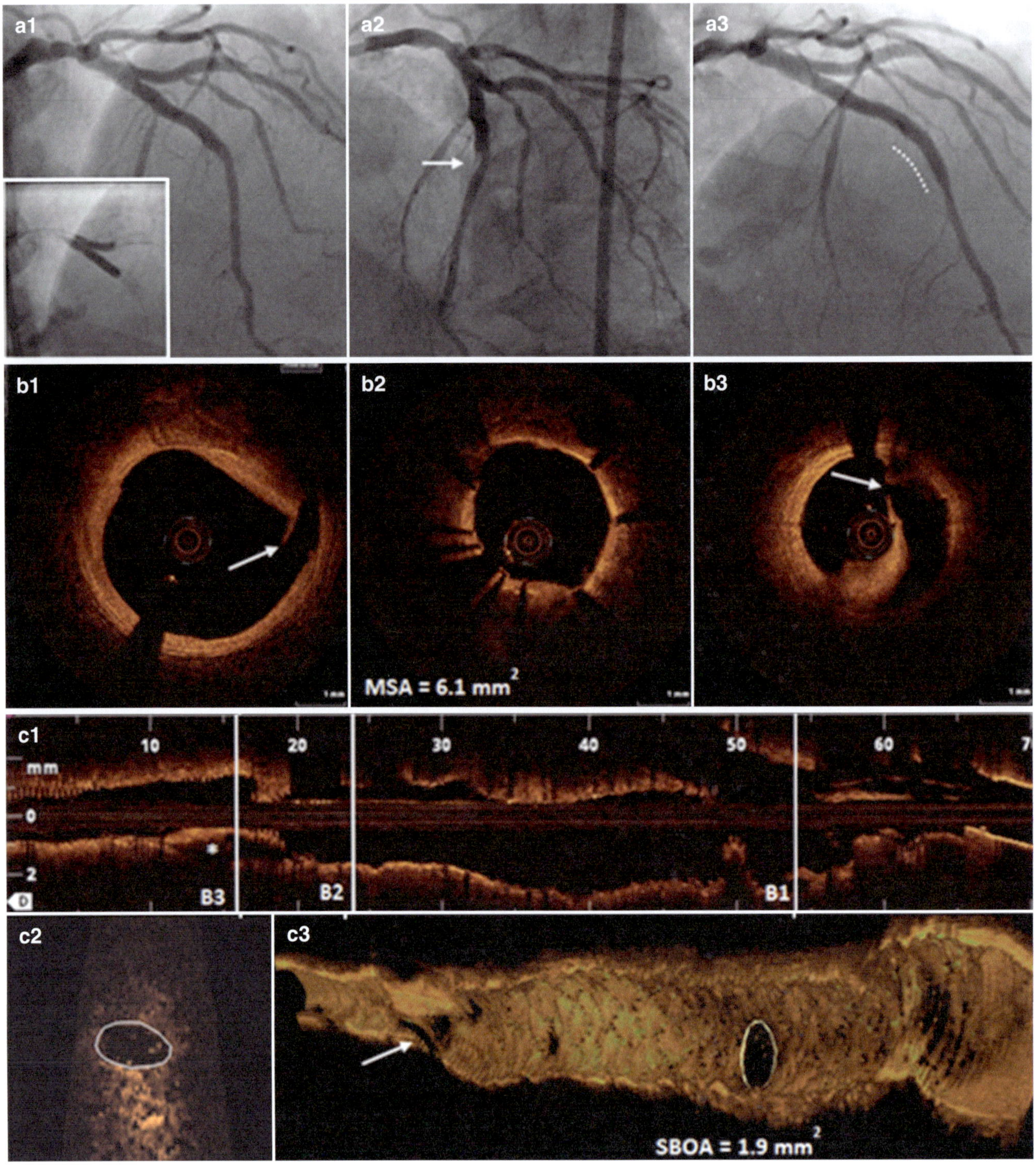

Fig. 3.15 After rotational atherectomy in the LAD with a 1.75 burr and in the first diagonal branch with a 1.25 mm burr, two everolimus-eluting platinum chromium stents were successfully implanted in the LAD and D1 (**a1**) using a modified T mini-crush stenting technique followed by final kissing balloon inflation (KBI) (**a1**, *inset*). Small distal edge dissection was visualized after stent deployment and KBI on angiogram (**a2**, *arrow*). OCT pullback of the main vessel showed well-apposed and expanded stent with the MSA of 6.1 mm^2 (**b2**), a 2-mm long proximal stent edge dissection (**b1**, *arrow*) and a larger 9 mm distal edge dissection (**b3**, *arrow*). The distal edge dissection can be visualized in the longitudinal OCT image (**c1**, *asterisk*). There was also a significant decrease in the SBOA from 3.8 to 1.9 mm^2 by three-dimensional OCT after stenting (**c2**, **c3**, *circled*). The *arrow* in **c3** points to a three-dimensional reconstruction of the distal stent edge dissection visualized by both angiography (**a2**) and OCT (**b3**). The distal dissection was successfully treated with an additional 3/12 mm DES (**a3**, *dotted line*) with no angiographically evident residual dissection. The present case highlights the utility of OCT in evaluating the immediate post-PCI complications in addition to selecting the most appropriate stenting strategy for bifurcation lesions

3.9 Case 8. OCT Guidance for Unprotected Left Main and LAD PCI: Looking Before Leaping in Treacherous Terrain (Figs. 3.16 and 3.17, Video 3.18)

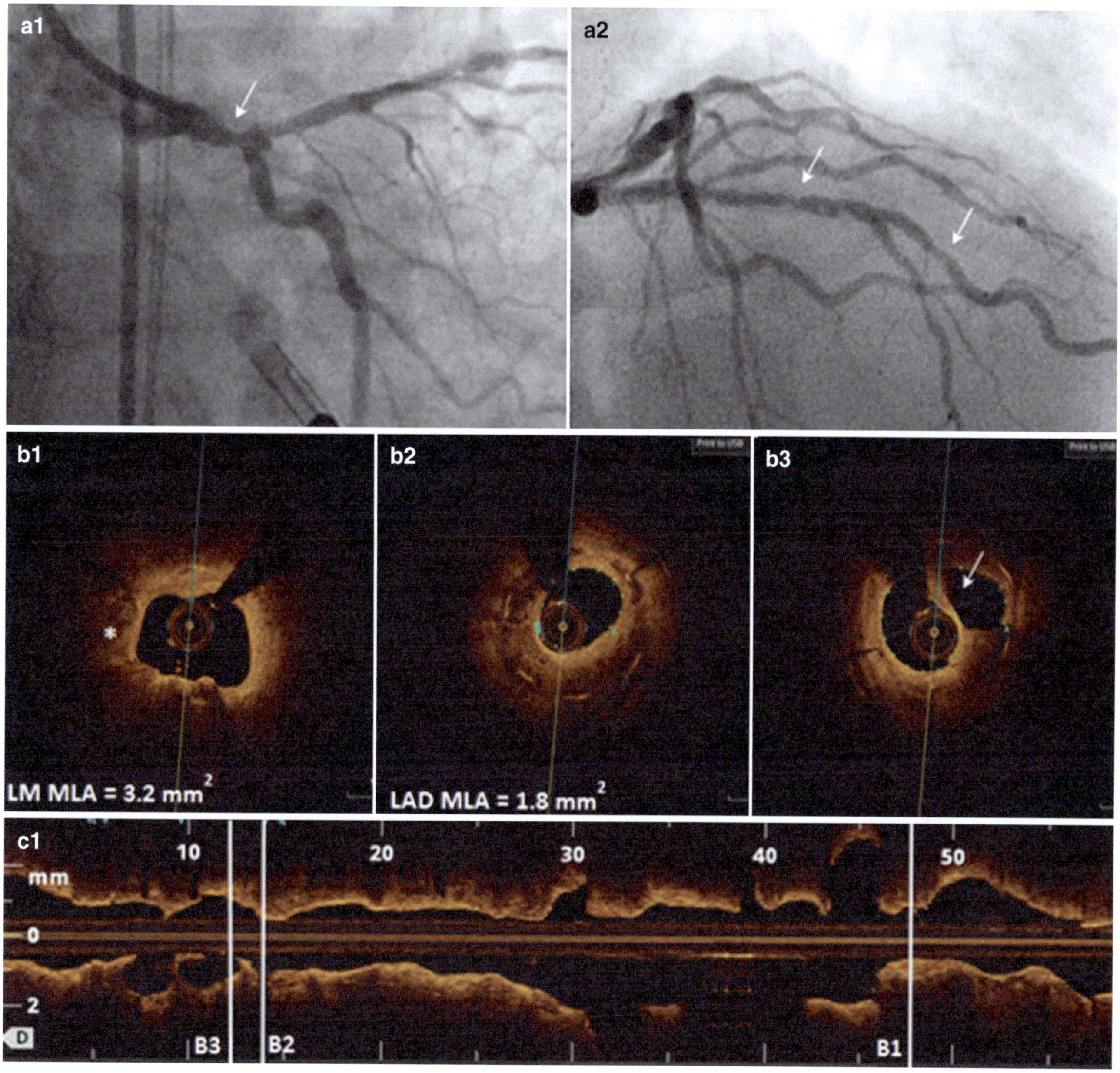

Fig. 3.16 Coronary angiography and OCT images before PCI. A 59-year-old male who was a smoker with hyperlipidemia, controlled hypertension, obesity, a prior history of MI, and chronic systolic heart failure presented with chest pain on mild exertion. A stress MPI scan showed an extensive area of moderate to severe partial ischemia with transient ischemic dilation of the left ventricle and severe systolic dysfunction. Coronary angiography showed a 70% stenosis of distal LM, 80% in-stent restenosis in the mid LAD, and 70% focal stenosis of distal LAD (**a1**, **a2**, *arrows*). OCT pullback of the LM and proximal LAD detected a focal calcified lesion in the left main (LM) with an MLA of 3.2 mm^2 (**b1**, *asterisk*) and an in-stent restenosis (ISR) lesion in the mid LAD with an MLA of 1.8 mm^2 (**b2**). A lipid-rich plaque with a healed neointimal plaque rupture was visualized inside the restenotic stent 2 mm distal to the MLA (**b3**, *arrow*)

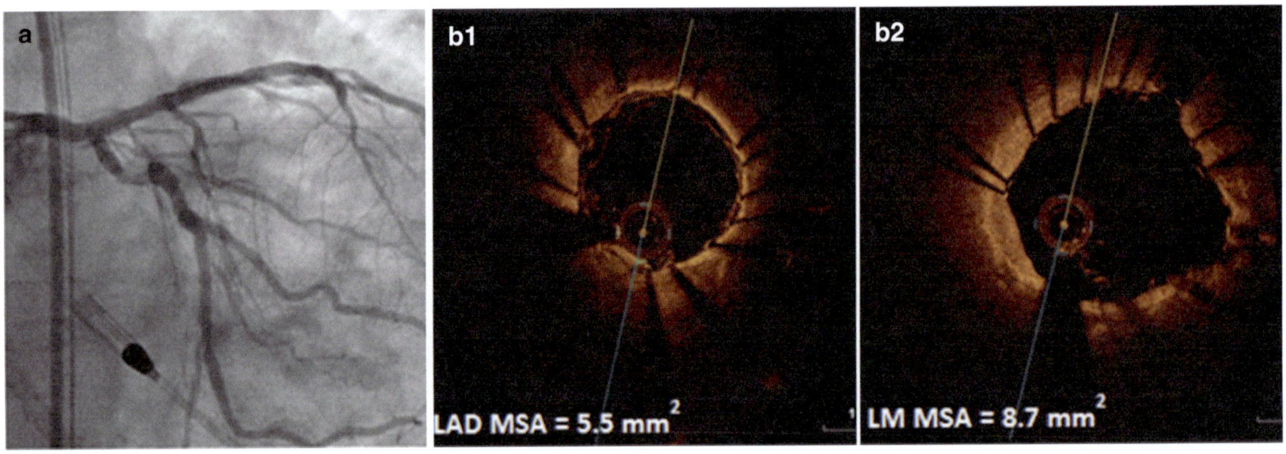

Fig. 3.17 Post-PCI angiogram and OCT images. After cutting balloon angioplasty, a 4/12-mm drug-eluting stent was deployed to cover the vessels from the mid LM to the proximal LAD; another 3/32 mm DES was placed in the mid LAD. The distal LAD was stented with a 2.5/24 mm DES after predilatation with a noncompliant balloon. After angiographically successful deployment of the stents (**a**), good stent apposition and expansion was confirmed by OCT imaging of the LM and proximal LAD (**b1**, **b2**)

3.10 Case 9. Severely Calcified Distal Left Main Bifurcation Lesion: On Cracking Tougher Nuts (Figs. 3.18 and 3.19, Videos 3.19 and 3.20)

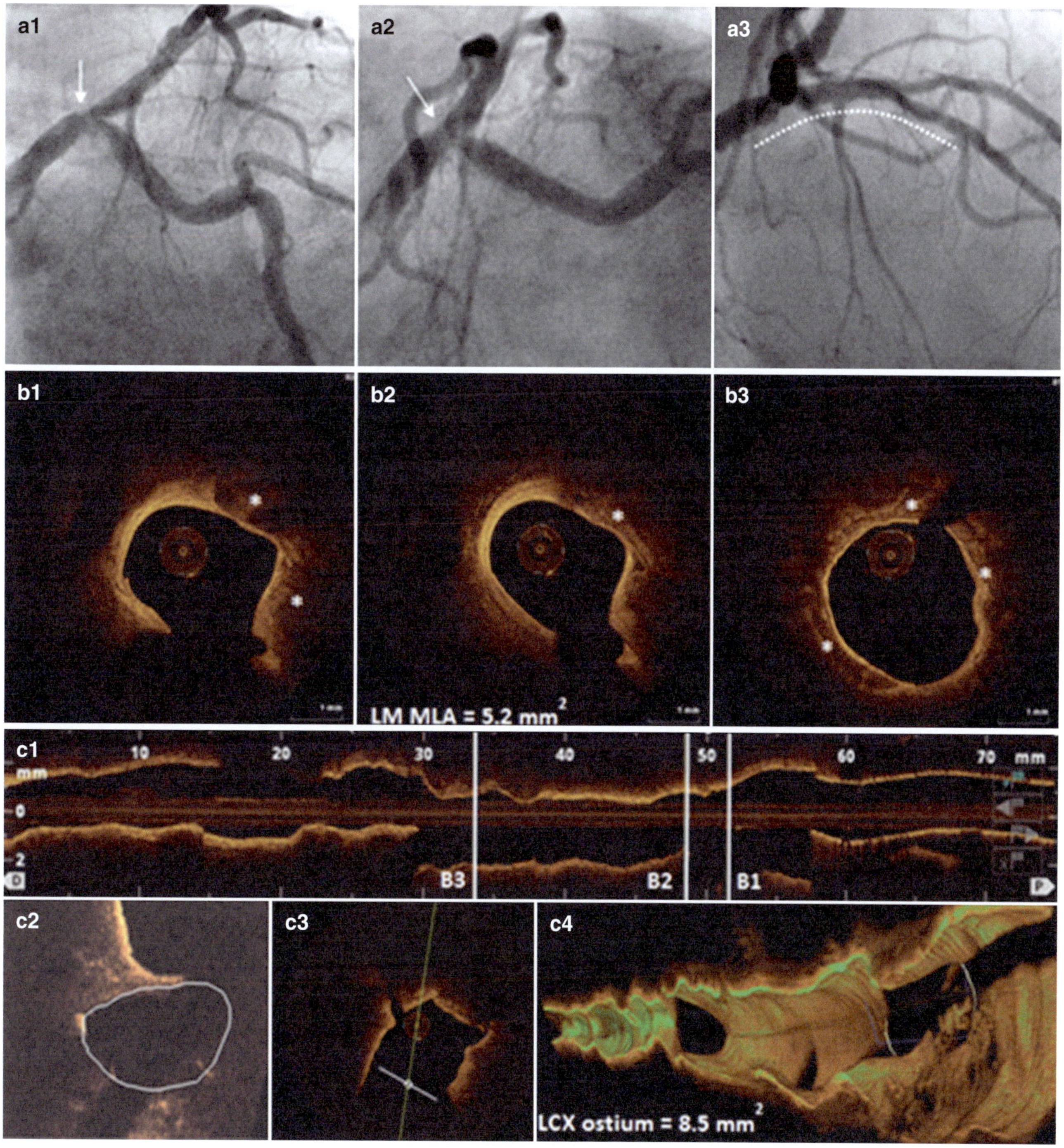

Fig. 3.18 Coronary angiography and OCT images. An 83-year-old female with known moderate left main disease since 2009 presented with a new onset of crescendo CCS Class III angina. A coronary angiogram revealed a calcified bifurcation lesion with 80% stenosis in the distal LM, 70% stenosis in the proximal LAD, and a 90% lesion in the proximal LCX (**a1**, **a2**, *arrows*). OCT imaging of the distal LM and proximal LAD (**a3**, *dotted line*) demonstrated significant stenosis in the distal LM with an MLA of 5.2 mm^2 (**b2**) and confirmed extensive calcification throughout the lesion, moderate calcification around the LM MLA site, (**b1**, **b2**, *asterisks*), and severe calcium in the LAD-D1 bifurcation area (**b3**, *asterisks*). The area of the LCX ostium before stenting was 8.5 mm^2 by three-dimensional OCT (**c2**–**c4**, *circled*)

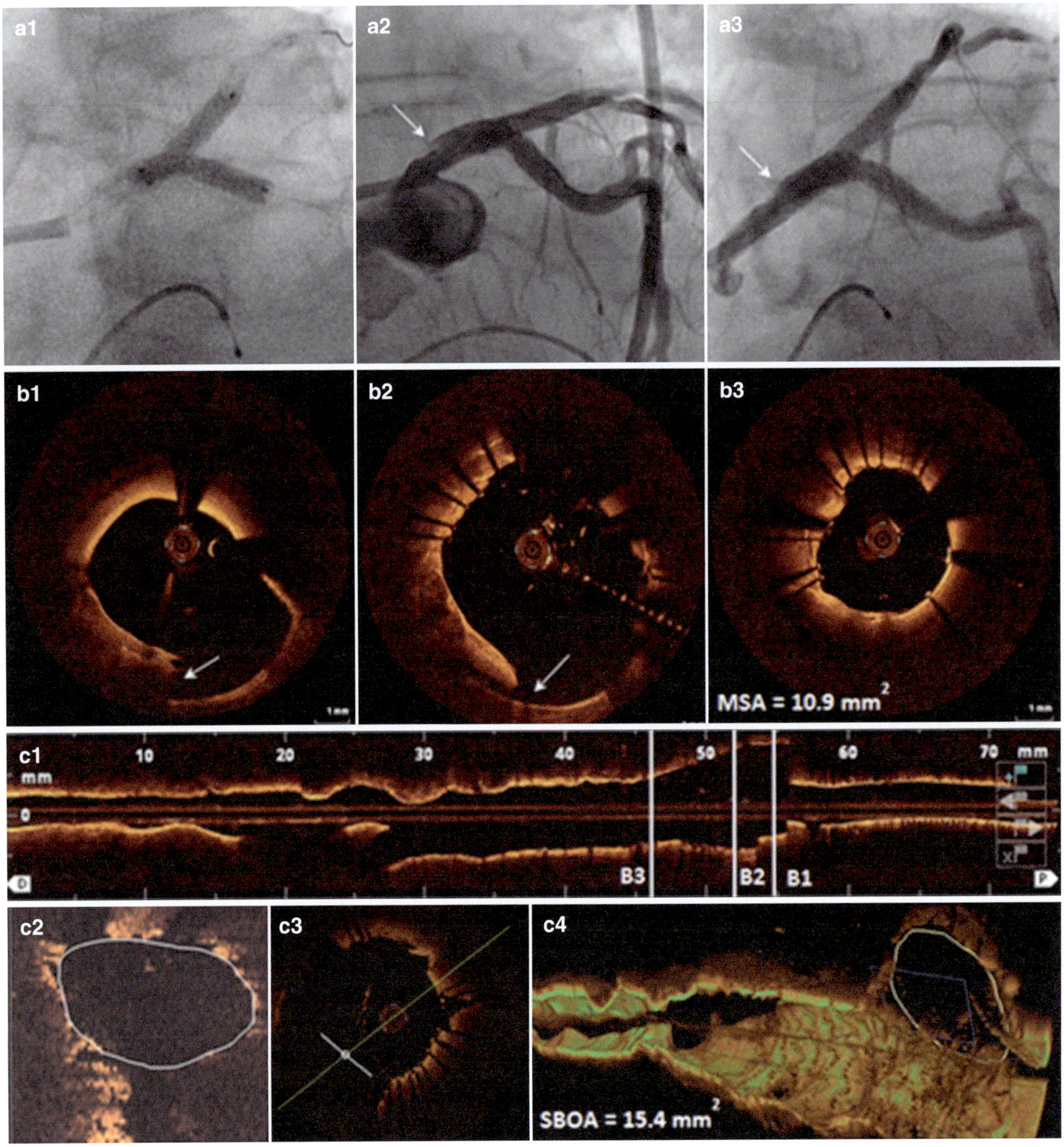

Fig. 3.19 Coronary angiography and OCT imaging after stenting. Rotational atherectomy was performed in the LCX, distal LM, and proximal LAD followed by a simultaneous kissing stents (SKSs) technique used for the LM-LAD bifurcation lesion with 4/15 mm everolimus eluting stents (**a1**). OCT confirmed good stent apposition and expansion of the LM/LAD stent with an MSA of 10.9 mm^2 (**b3**). The ostial LCx lumen area after stenting increased to 15.4 mm^2 (**c2–c4**). A non–flow limiting type B dissection proximal to the stents was noted on the angiogram (**a2**, *arrow*) and detected by OCT (**b1**, **b2**, *arrow*). The dissection was classified as a medial dissection at the proximal edge of the stent with a length of 3.6 mm. Two additional 4/8 mm everolimus eluting stents were deployed overlapping the initial stents using the SKS technique; the final KBI was performed with stent balloons. There was a small residual dissection on angiogram unchanged during 15 min of observation (**a3**)

3.11 Case 10. Periprocedural Myocardial Infarction After Proximal RCA PCI: On Predicting Inclement Weather (Figs. 3.20 and 3.21, Videos 3.21 and 3.22)

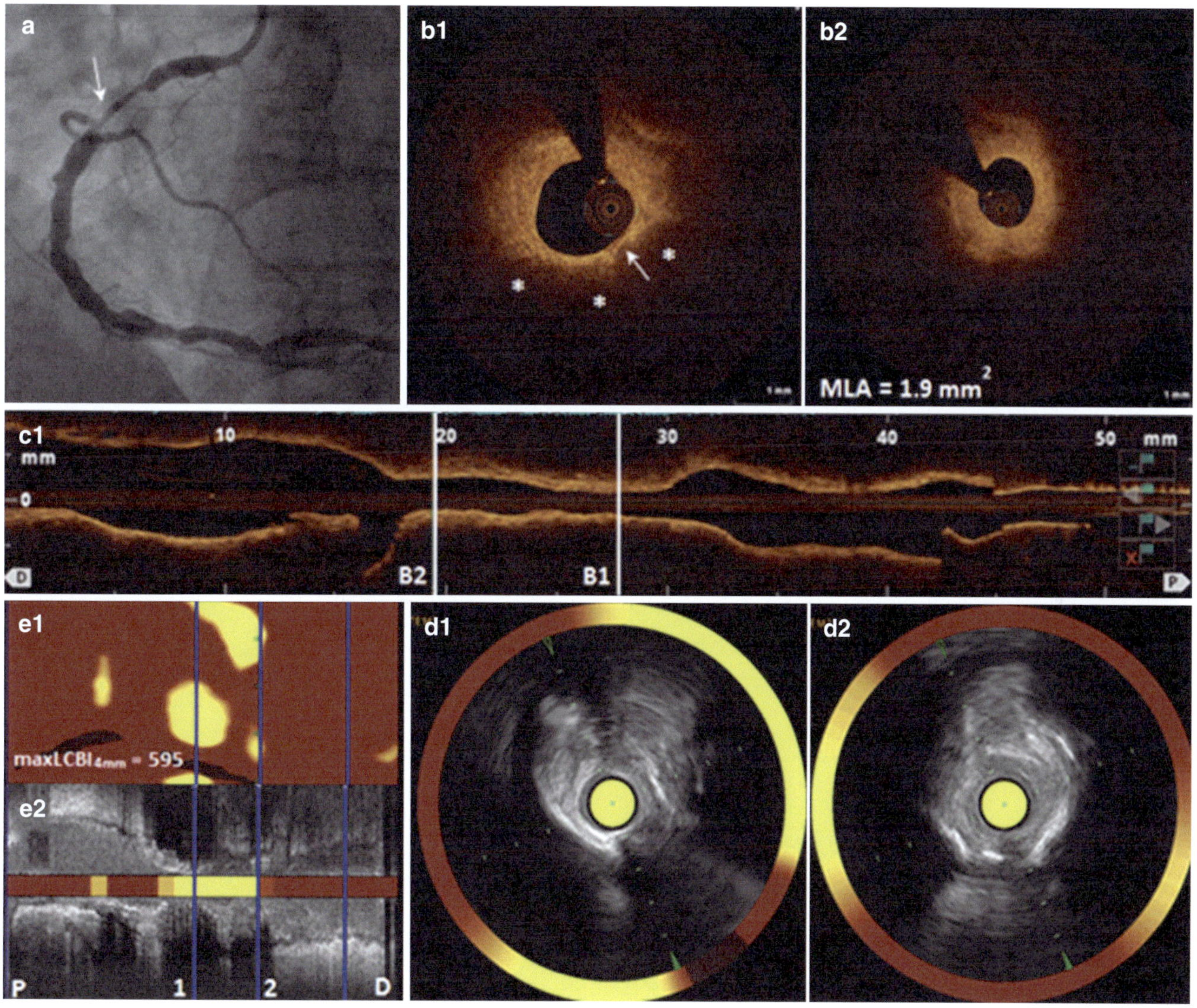

Fig. 3.20 Coronary angiography and intravascular imaging before stenting. A 57-year-old male with controlled hypertension and hyperlipidemia presented with CCS class III angina and high-risk findings on SPECT MPI. The patient had an 80–90% proximal RCA lesion on coronary angiogram (**a**, *arrow*). OCT and combined IVUS/NIRS imaging performed in the same segment detected a lesion with an MLA of 1.9 and 2.5 mm² by OCT and IVUS, respectively (**b2**, **d2**). OCT revealed a large lipid-rich plaque (*asterisks*) with the minimal cap thickness of 60 µm (*arrow*) proximal to the MLA site (**b1**), the corresponding IVUS cross-sectional image in shown in D1. Preintervention NIRS demonstrated a large yellow plaque occupying more than 50% of the vessel circumference with a $maxLCBI_{4mm}$ of 595 (**e1**, **e2**)

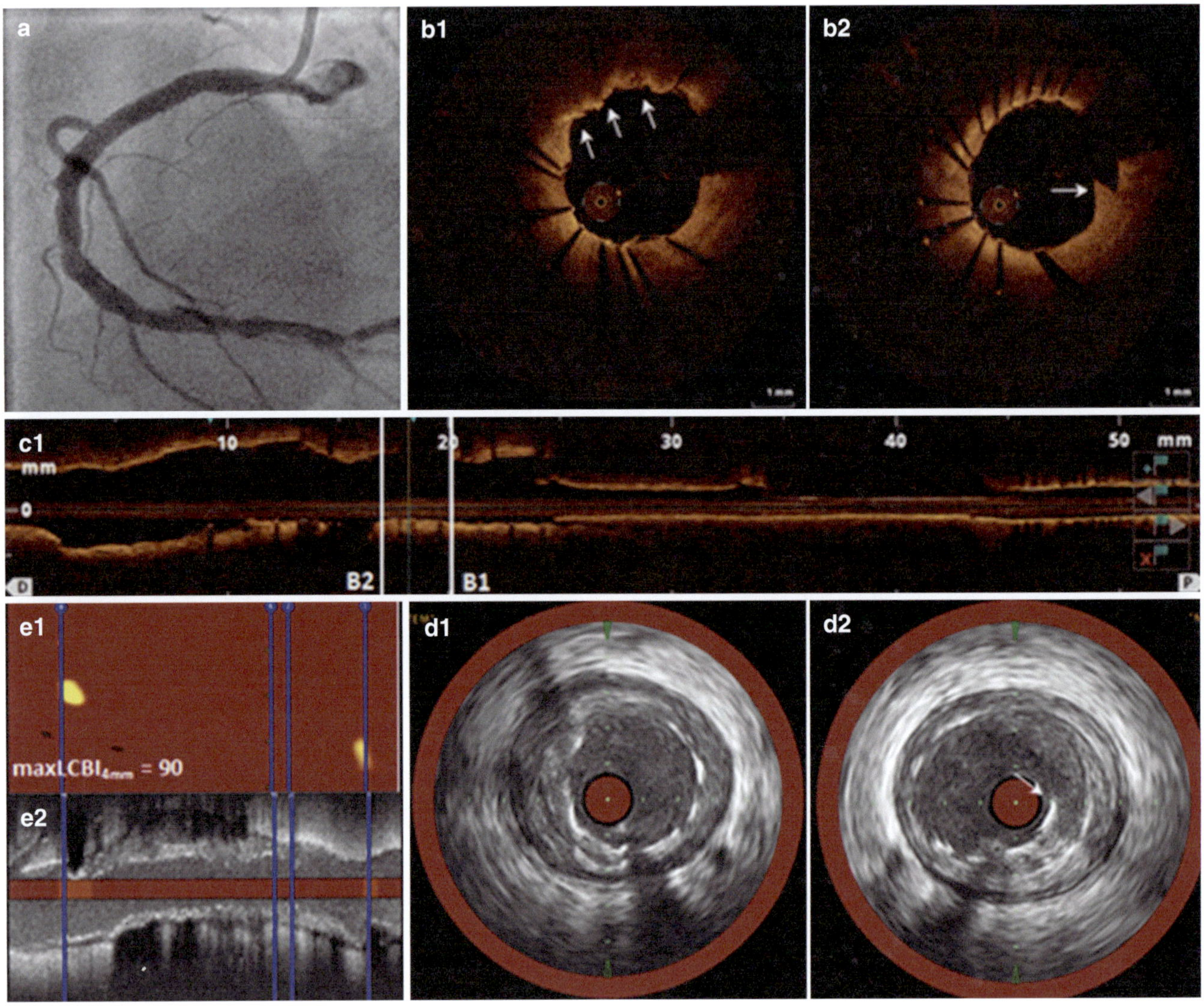

Fig. 3.21 Postintervention angiogram, OCT, and IVUS/NIRS imaging. A 4/20-mm stent was successfully deployed in the proximal RCA (**a**); there was a transient slow flow observed after stenting. Postintervention NIRS revealed almost complete disappearance of the lipid-rich yellow plaque, maxLCBI4mm = 90 (**e1**, **e2**). Good stent apposition and expansion were confirmed by OCT (**b1**, **b2**) and IVUS (**d1**, **d2**). Soft plaque protrusion was detected by OCT around the MLA (**b1**, *arrows*) and small intimal dissection was visualized by both OCT (**b2**, *arrow*) and IVUS (**d2**, *arrow*). Despite excellent angiographic and intravascular imaging outcomes of stenting, the patient developed post-procedural myocardial infarction with elevation of cardiac troponin I (cTnI) level (4.5 ng/mL) within 24 h of PCI

References

1. Tsuchida K, van der Giessen WJ, Patterson M, Tanimoto S, Garcia-Garcia H, Regar E, et al. In vivo validation of a novel three-dimensional quantitative coronary angiography system (CardiOp-B): comparison with a conventional two-dimensional system (CAAS II) and with special reference to optical coherence tomography. EuroIntervention. 2007;3:100–8.
2. Okamura T, Onuma Y, Garcia-Garcia HM, van Geuns RJ, Wykrzykowska JJ, Schultz C, et al. First-in-man evaluation of intravascular optical frequency domain imaging (OFDI) of Terumo: a comparison with intravascular ultrasound and quantitative coronary angiography. EuroIntervention. 2011;6:1037–45.
3. Okamura T, Gonzalo N, Gutierrez-Chico JL, Serruys PW, Bruining N, de Winter S, et al. Reproducibility of coronary Fourier domain optical coherence tomography: quantitative analysis of in vivo stented coronary arteries using three different software packages. EuroIntervention. 2010;6:371–9.
4. Fedele S, Biondi-Zoccai G, Kwiatkowski P, Di Vito L, Occhipinti M, Cremonesi A, et al. Reproducibility of coronary optical coherence tomography for lumen and length measurements in humans (The CLI-VAR [Centro per la Lotta contro l'Infarto-VARiability] study). Am J Cardiol. 2012;110:1106–12.
5. Sihan K, Botha C, Post F, de Winter S, Gonzalo N, Regar E, et al. Fully automatic three-dimensional quantitative analysis of intracoronary optical coherence tomography: method and Validation. Catheter Cardiovasc Interv. 2009;74:1058–65.
6. Tanimoto S, Rodriguez-Granillo G, Barlis P, de Winter S, Bruining N, Hamers R, et al. A novel approach for quantitative analysis of intracoronary optical coherence tomography: high inter-observer agreement with computer-assisted contour detection. Catheter Cardiovasc Interv. 2008;72:228–35.
7. Kini AS, Baber U, Kovacic JC, Limaye A, Ali ZA, Sweeny J, et al. Changes in plaque lipid content after short-term intensive versus standard statin therapy: the YELLOW trial (reduction in yellow plaque by aggressive lipid-lowering therapy). J Am Coll Cardiol. 2013;62:21–9.
8. Tomey MI, Sharma SK. Interventional options for coronary artery calcification. Curr Cardiol Rep. 2016;18:12.
9. Al Suwaidi J, Berger PB, Rihal CS, Garratt KN, Bell MR, Ting HH, et al. Immediate and long-term outcome of intracoronary stent implantation for true bifurcation lesions. J Am Coll Cardiol. 2000;35:929–36.
10. Lakovou I, Ge L, Colombo A. Contemporary stent treatment of coronary bifurcations. J Am Coll Cardiol. 2005;46:1446–55.
11. Maeng M, Holm NR, Erglis A, Kumsars I, Niemelä M, Kervinen K, et al. Long-term results after simple versus complex stenting of coronary artery bifurcation lesions: Nordic Bifurcation Study 5-year follow-up results. J Am Coll Cardiol. 2013;62:30–4.
12. Farooq V, Serruys PW, Heo JH, Gogas BD, Okamura T, Gomez-Lara J, et al. New insights into the coronary artery bifurcation hypothesis-generating concepts utilizing 3-dimensional optical frequency domain imaging. JACC Cardiovasc Interv. 2011;4:921–31.
13. Kini AS, Yoshimura T, Vengrenyuk Y, Amirian J, Hasan C, Baber U, et al. Plaque morphology predictors of side branch occlusion after main vessel stenting in coronary bifurcation lesions: optical coherence tomography imaging study. JACC Cardiovasc Interv. 2016;9:862–5.
14. Kini AS, Vengrenyuk Y, Pena J, Yoshimura T, Panwar SR, Motoyama S, et al. Plaque morphology predictors of side branch occlusion after provisional stenting in coronary bifurcation lesion: results of optical coherence tomography bifurcation study (ORBID). Catheter Cardiovasc Interv. 2017;89(2):259–68. doi:10.1002/ccd.26524.
15. Serruys PW, Morice MC, Kappetein AP, Colombo A, Holmes DR, Mack MJ, et al. Percutaneous coronary intervention versus coronary-artery bypass grafting for severe coronary artery disease. N Engl J Med. 2009;360:961–72.
16. Alam M, Huang HD, Shahzad SA, Kar B, Virani SS, Rogers PA, et al. Percutaneous coronary intervention vs. coronary artery bypass graft surgery for unprotected left main coronary artery disease in the drug-eluting stents era—an aggregate data meta-analysis of 11,148 patients. Circ J. 2013;77:372–82.
17. Fujino Y, Bezerra HG, Attizzani GF, Wang W, Yamamoto H, Chamié D, et al. Frequency-domain optical coherence tomography assessment of unprotected left main coronary artery disease-a comparison with intravascular ultrasound. Catheter Cardiovasc Interv. 2013;82:E173–83.
18. Lee T, Yonetsu T, Koura K, Hishikari K, Murai T, Iwai T, et al. Impact of coronary plaque morphology assessed by optical coherence tomography on cardiac troponin elevation in patients with elective stent implantation. Circ Cardiovasc Interv. 2011;4:378–86.
19. Porto I, Di Vito L, Burzotta F, Niccoli G, Trani C, Leone AM, et al. Predictors of periprocedural (type IVa) myocardial infarction, as assessed by frequency-domain optical coherence tomography. Circ Cardiovasc Interv. 2012;5:89–96, S1–6.
20. Kini AS, Motoyama S, Vengrenyuk Y, Feig JE, Pena J, Baber U, et al. Multimodality intravascular imaging to predict periprocedural myocardial infarction during percutaneous coronary intervention. JACC Cardiovasc Interv. 2015;8:937–45.

Post-Stent Evaluation, Stent Thrombosis, and In-Stent Restenosis

4

4.1 Introduction

Optimization of stent deployment during percutaneous coronary interventions (PCI) is one of the most important factors in achieving favorable immediate and long-term outcomes. Intravascular ultrasound (IVUS) imaging studies demonstrated that the strongest predictor of early stent thrombosis and restenosis is the absolute degree of stent expansion characterized by the minimal stent area (MSA) after PCI [1, 2]. Stent underexpansion is poorly recognized by angiography. By achieving greater stent expansion, IVUS-guided PCI has been associated with significant reduction in the risk of major adverse coronary events (MACE) compared to angiography-guided PCI [3].

Although optical coherence tomography (OCT) has higher resolution compared to IVUS, the limited penetration depth by OCT does not allow visualization of the external elastic membrane (EEM) and assessment of the vessel size, an important measurement used in IVUS-guided trials. Whether OCT-guidance can result in a similar degree of stent expansion compared to IVUS-guided PCI has been under investigation by a series of ILUMIEN trials. In a *post hoc* analysis of two prospective imaging trials (ILUMIEN II), IVUS and OCT guidance demonstrated a comparable degree of stent expansion [4]. Post-PCI MSA with OCT guidance was non-inferior to that of IVUS-guidance in the first prospective randomized trial, ILUMIEN III. Procedural and 30 day MACE were also similar between the groups [5]. The goal of the next randomized study, ILUMIEN IV, is to determine whether similar clinical outcomes can be obtained after stenting guided by these imaging modalities.

In addition to stent underexpansion, OCT can detect several features of suboptimal stent deployment including edge dissection, malapposition, intrastent plaque protrusion, and reference lumen area narrowing. In-stent minimum lumen area less than 4.5 mm^2, distal stent edge dissection more than 200 μm, and the reference lumen area less than 4.5 mm^2 at either distal or proximal stent edge were independent predictors of MACE in a retrospective analysis with 1 year follow-up [6]. In contrast, percent stent expansion less than 70%, stent malapposition more than 200 μm, large plaque protrusion and proximal edge dissection more than 200 μm, were not associated with worse clinical outcomes. Multiple reports emphasize the importance of adequate high pressure post-dilatation to obtain optimal stent expansion in order to reduce the risks of complications [7]. It is important to select a technique that allows for avoidance of unwanted and potentially dangerous complications caused by vessel overstretching. Postdilatation with noncompliant balloons has been shown to improve MSA without causing deeper injury of the vessel wall with intima-media rupture [7].

Stent thrombosis (ST) is an infrequent but highly morbid complication of PCI with mortality rates of 10–20% during the first year [8, 9]. PCI for ST is associated with a low rate of reperfusion and high rates of recurrent ST, myocardial infarction (MI), and death [10–12]. Unfavorable long-term outcomes with a high mortality and ST recurrence rate of 26% were observed after a first definite ST [9]. Premature discontinuation of antiplatelet therapy, renal failure, bifurcation lesion PCI, diabetes, and low ejection fraction were identified as predictors of future thrombotic events [13]. Procedure-related factors including stent underexpansion and residual reference segment stenosis have been shown to play a major role in early ST, which occurs within 1 month of stent implantation [14, 15]. Impaired re-endothelialization, incomplete stent apposition or fracture, hypersensitivity to the drug-eluting stent (DES) polymer, chronic inflammation with outward remodeling, and neoatherosclerotic plaque rupture play important roles in late (1–12 month after stent implantation) and very late ST (more than 12 month after stenting) [16, 17]. Increased risk of ST is also associated with inadequate antiplatelet therapy and/or resistance to antiplatelet treatment [18, 19]. OCT imaging represents a unique tool for ST diagnosis and evaluation. It can help understand

Electronic Supplementary Material The online version of this chapter (doi:10.1007/978-3-319-62666-6_4) contains supplementary material, which is available to authorized users.

A. Kini et al., *Atlas of Coronary Intravascular Optical Coherence Tomography*, DOI 10.1007/978-3-319-62666-6_4

whether a procedure-related mechanism is involved in ST and select the most appropriate treatment strategy. Stent underexpansion and strut malapposition are the most common procedural factors leading to ST. In addition, the length of the segment with uncovered struts by OCT was an independent predictor of late stent thrombosis after DES implantation [17]. Therefore, efforts should be made to ensure optimal stent expansion and apposition after stenting. OCT can help identify and correct suboptimal stent implantation, which can prevent ST recurrence in future.

Although introduction of DES dramatically reduced the occurrence of aggressive neointimal proliferation, treatment of in-stent restenosis (ISR) after stent implantation remains a major clinical problem [20]. Treatment of patients with ISR lesions includes conventional coronary balloon angioplasty (BA), cutting and scoring balloon therapy, stenting, atherectomy, and vascular brachytherapy. Intrastent plaque morphology assessment with OCT imaging can positively impact outcomes by optimizing PCI in complex lesions. OCT imaging can provide unique insights into the underlying substrates of ISR by detailed visualization of neointimal tissue and select the best treatment strategy for the patient and to make the decision whether another stent implantation is necessary. While normal neointimal tissue in DES mainly consists of smooth muscle cells and extracellular matrix, recent pathological and imaging studies provided convincing evidence for the presence of atherosclerosis within stent neointima, or neoatherosclerosis [21–24]. Neoatherosclerosis is characterized by neointimal formation of lipid-rich plaque and calcification and may represent an important mechanism of DES failure. OCT imaging can provide unique insights into the etiology of in-stent restenosis and help select the most appropriate treatment strategy. Rotational atherectomy has been successfully used in calcified neoatherosclerosis causing undilatable in-stent restenosis [25, 26]. In addition, OCT imaging before stenting can assess the risks for periprocedural myocardial infarction. The unstable features of neoatherosclerosis including thin-cap fibroatheroma and plaque rupture were the most common findings in patients with periprocedural myocardial infarction [27].

4.2 Case 1. Stent Malapposition (Figs. 4.1, 4.2 and 4.3, Videos 4.1, 4.2 and 4.3)

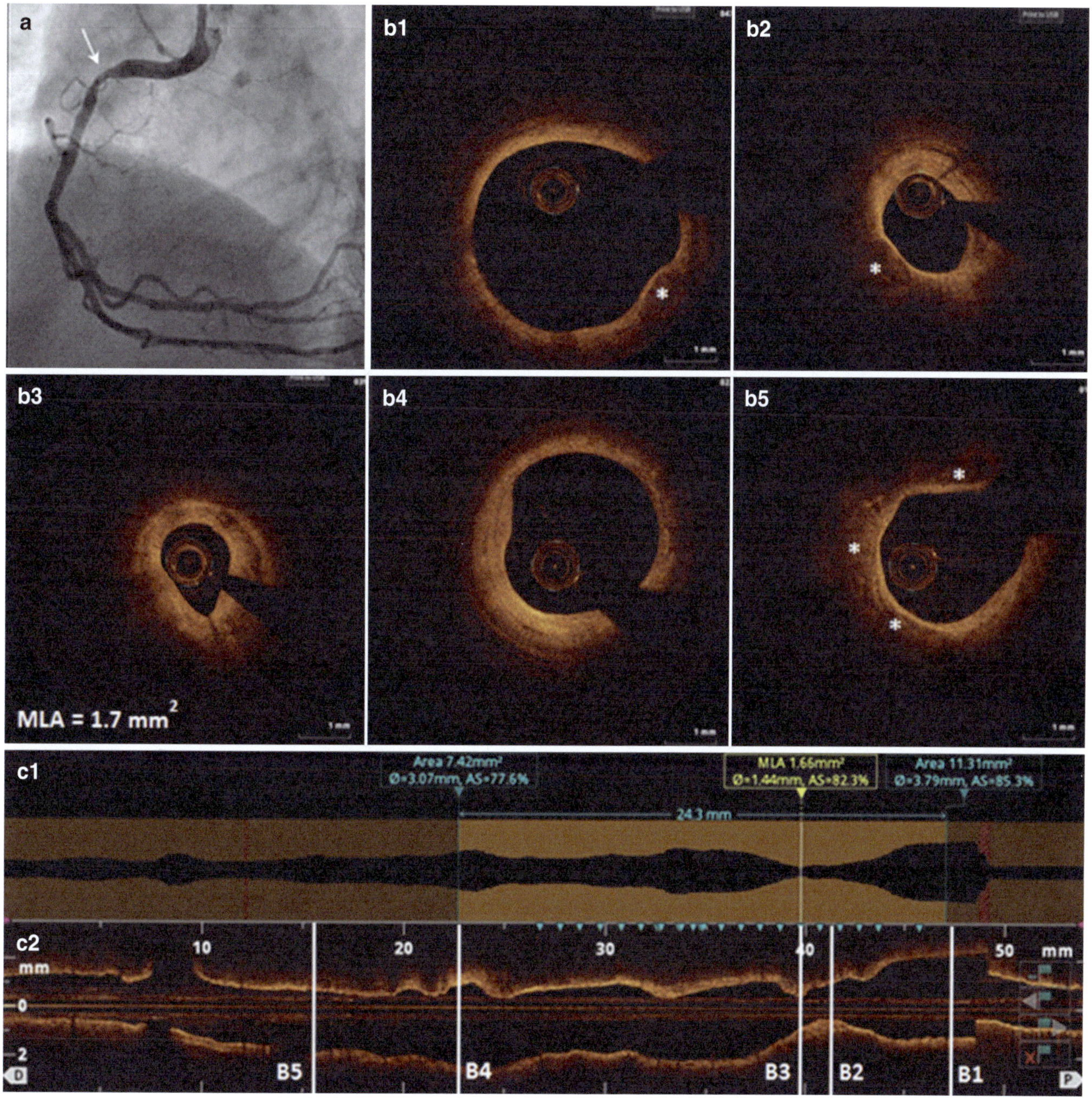

Fig. 4.1 Coronary angiography and OCT imaging before percutaneous coronary intervention (PCI). A 73-year-old female, ex-smoker, with controlled non-insulin dependent diabetes mellitus (NIDDM), hyperlipidemia and hypertension presented for staged PCI of the RCA. Angiography demonstrated 80–90% eccentric lesion in the proximal RCA (**a**, *arrow*). OCT automatic lumen profile feature (**c1**) was used to assess the degree of stenosis (82.3%), references, and plaque morphology. OCT imaging detected fibrocalcific plaque with spotty (less than one quadrant) calcification proximal to MLA (**b2**, *asterisk*), and minimal disease at the proximal (**b1**) and distal (**b4**) reference sites with 3 and 3.8 mm lumen diameters respectively. Another spotty calcification was visualized at the proximal reference site (**b1**, asterisk). Severe (three-quadrant) calcification was detected distal to the lesion (**b5**, *asterisks*). Based on the lesion assessment by OCT, a 3.5/23 mm drug eluting stent (DES) was selected for the lesion and implanted after predilatation with a noncompliant balloon

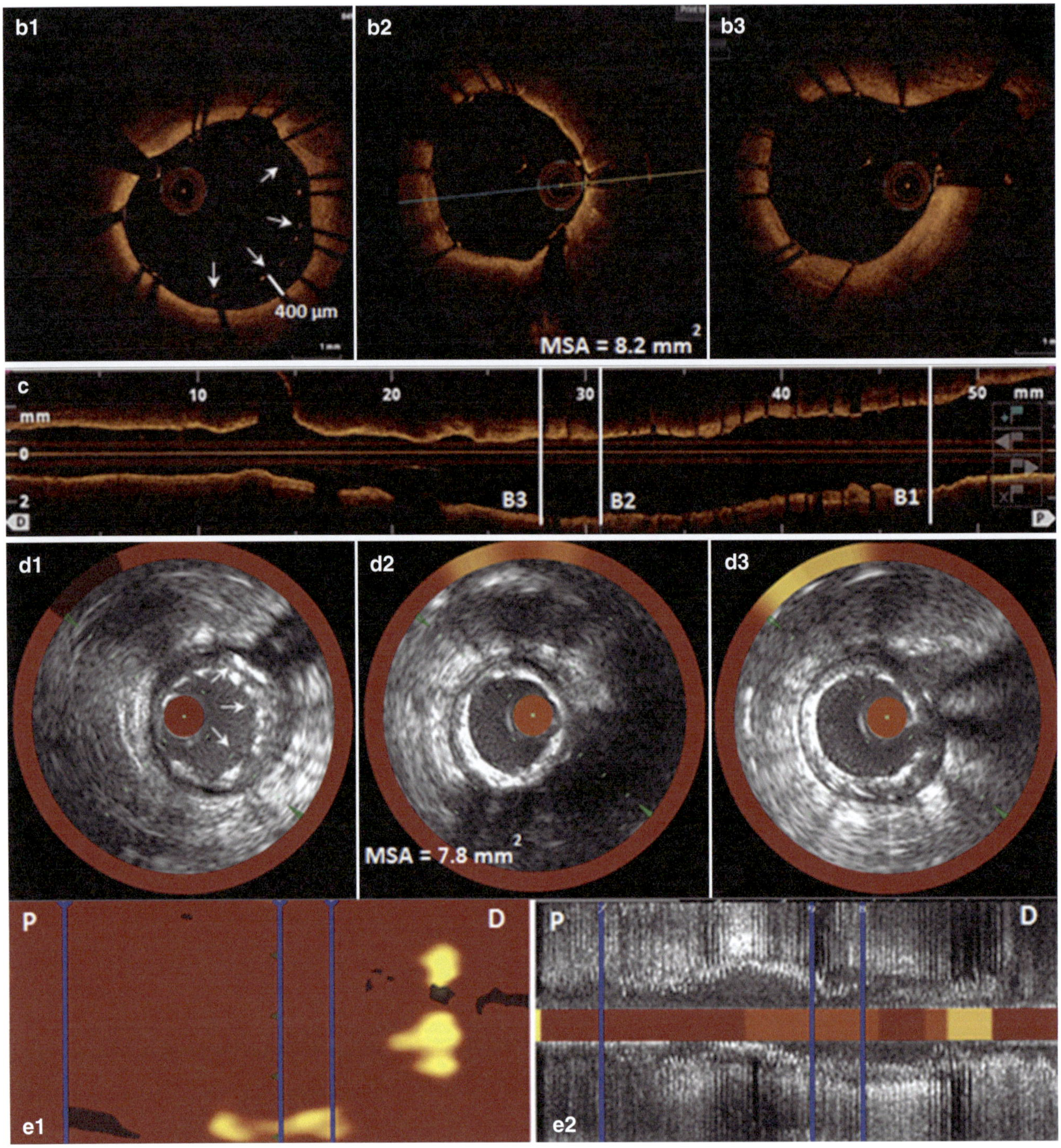

Fig. 4.2 OCT and intravascular ultrasound (IVUS)/near infrared spectroscopy (NIRS) images after stenting. Large circumferential stent malapposition was detected by OCT at the proximal edge of the stent with maximal malapposition distance of 400 μm (**b**1, *arrows*). The lumen and stent areas in the frame were measured 11.4 and 8.7 mm^2 respectively. MSA of 8.2 mm^2 suggested good stent expansion (**b2**); there was no malapposition or dissection detected at the distal edge of the stent (**b3**). In addition to OCT, IVUS/NIRS imaging of the same lesion was performed (**d1**–**d3**, **e1**, **e2**). The MSA location was detected by IVUS manually (**d2**). IVUS crosssections (**d1**) and (**d3**) correspond to the OCT frames (**b1**) and (**b3**). OCT image of the proximal stent edge (**b1**) provides more clear visualization of stent malapposition compared with IVUS (**d1**). Stent postdilatation was performed with a 4/12 mm noncompliant balloon at 18 atm

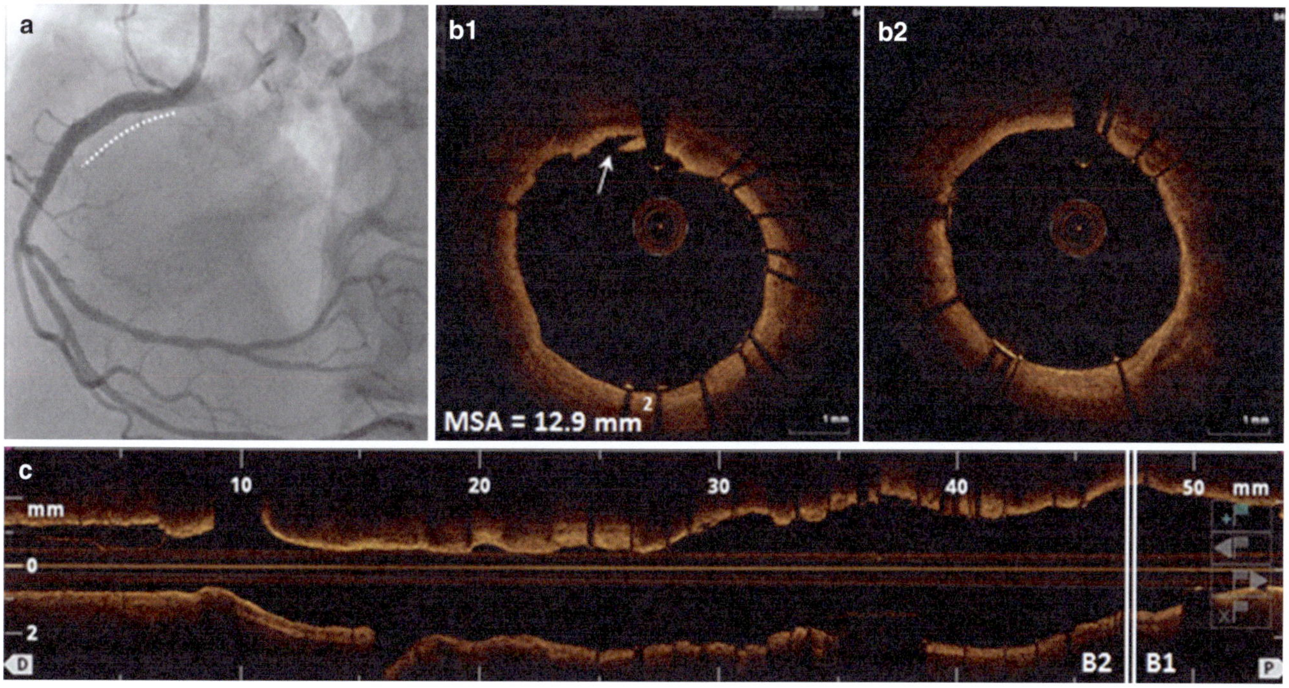

Fig. 4.3 Final post-PCI coronary angiography and OCT images. Proximal stent malapposition was resolved after postdilatation (**b1**, **b2**). Maximal stent area increased from 8.7 to 12.9 mm^2 and was detected at the proximal edge of the stent (**b1**). A small intimal in-stent dissection was visualized after postdilatation at the site of MSA (**b1**, *arrow*). In this case, detection of large circumferential stent malapposition by OCT imaging led to postdilatation with a noncompliant balloon, which resulted in resolved strut malapposition and minimal tissue injury

4.3 Case 2. Stent Malapposition and Underexpansion (Figs. 4.4, 4.5 and 4.6, Videos 4.4, 4.5 and 4.6)

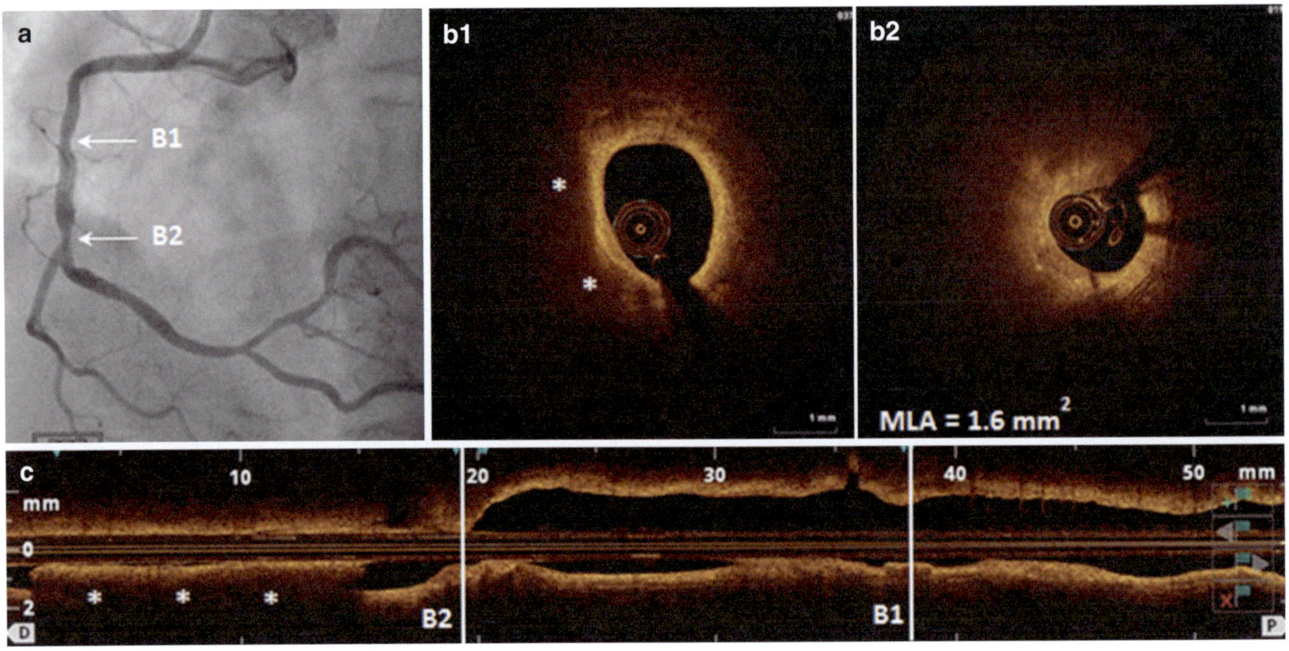

Fig. 4.4 Coronary angiography and OCT imaging before PCI. A 62-year-old female, ex-smoker with controlled hypertension and hyperlipidemia presented with CCS Class III angina, shortness of breath with minimal exertion, and ischemic ECG change on stress echocardiography. Coronary angiography showed a 70–80% stenosis and a nonocclusive lesion in the proximal part of the vessel (**a**, *arrows*). OCT detected two focal stenoses with lumen area of 3.14 (**b1**) and 1.6 mm^2 (**b2**). There was no calcification detected by OCT in the segment; a lipid-rich (**b1**, *asterisks*) and mostly fibrous (**b2**) plaques were visualized at the site of stenoses. The distal portion of the OCT pullback was not analyzable due to insufficient blood clearance (**c**, *asterisks*). A 3/32 mm everolimus eluting stent was selected for the lesion in order to cover both stenoses

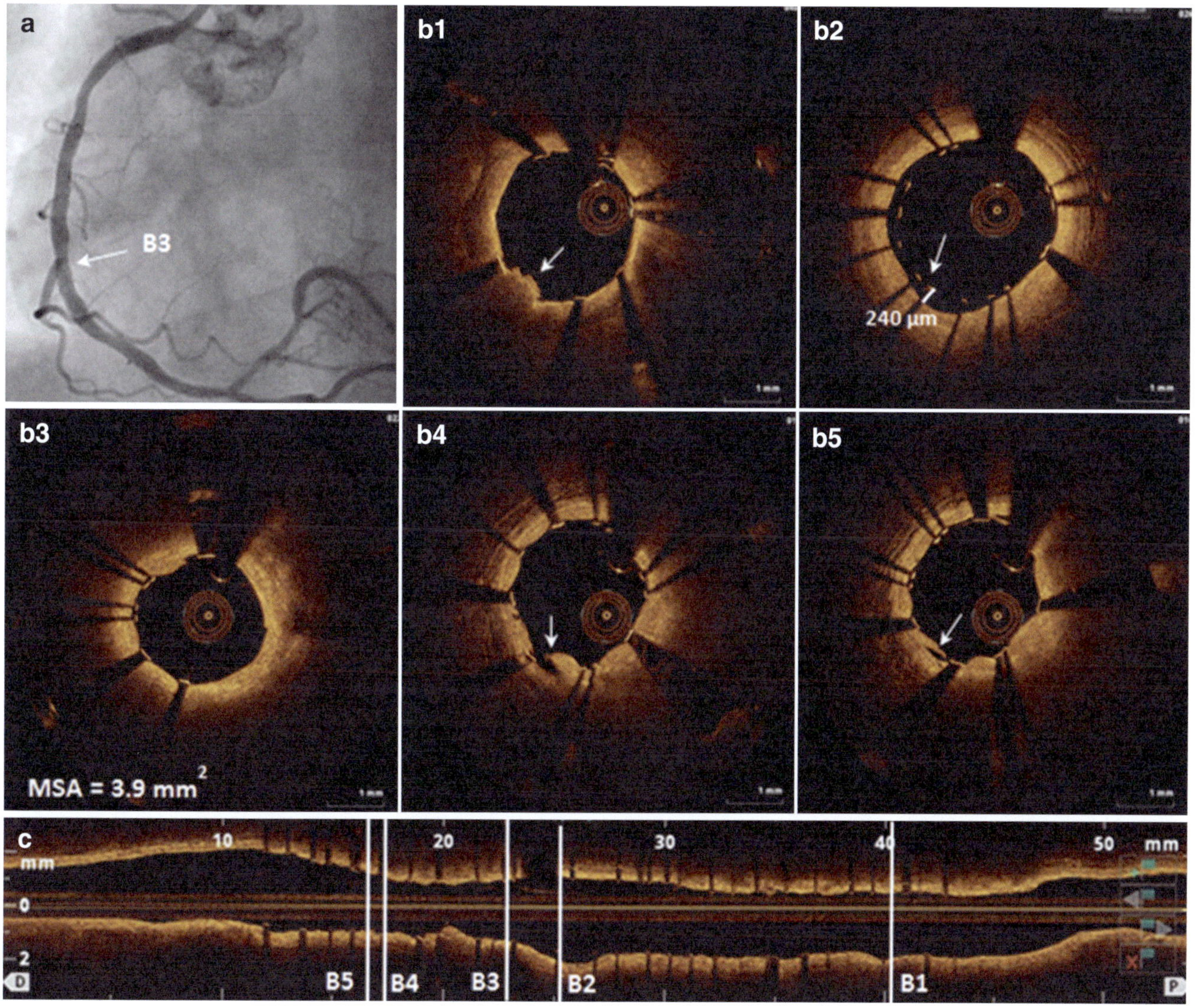

Fig. 4.5 Coronary angiogram and OCT imaging after stenting. OCT after stent implantation detected stent underexpansion with MSA of 3.9 mm^2 (**b3**). In addition, OCT visualized a proximal plaque protrusion (**b1**), stent malapposition with the largest distance of 240 µm (**b2**, *arrow*), and small intimal in-stent dissections at the distal portion of the stent (**b4**, **b5**, *arrow*). Based on the imaging findings, postdilatation was performed with a 3/20 mm noncompliant balloon at 18 atm

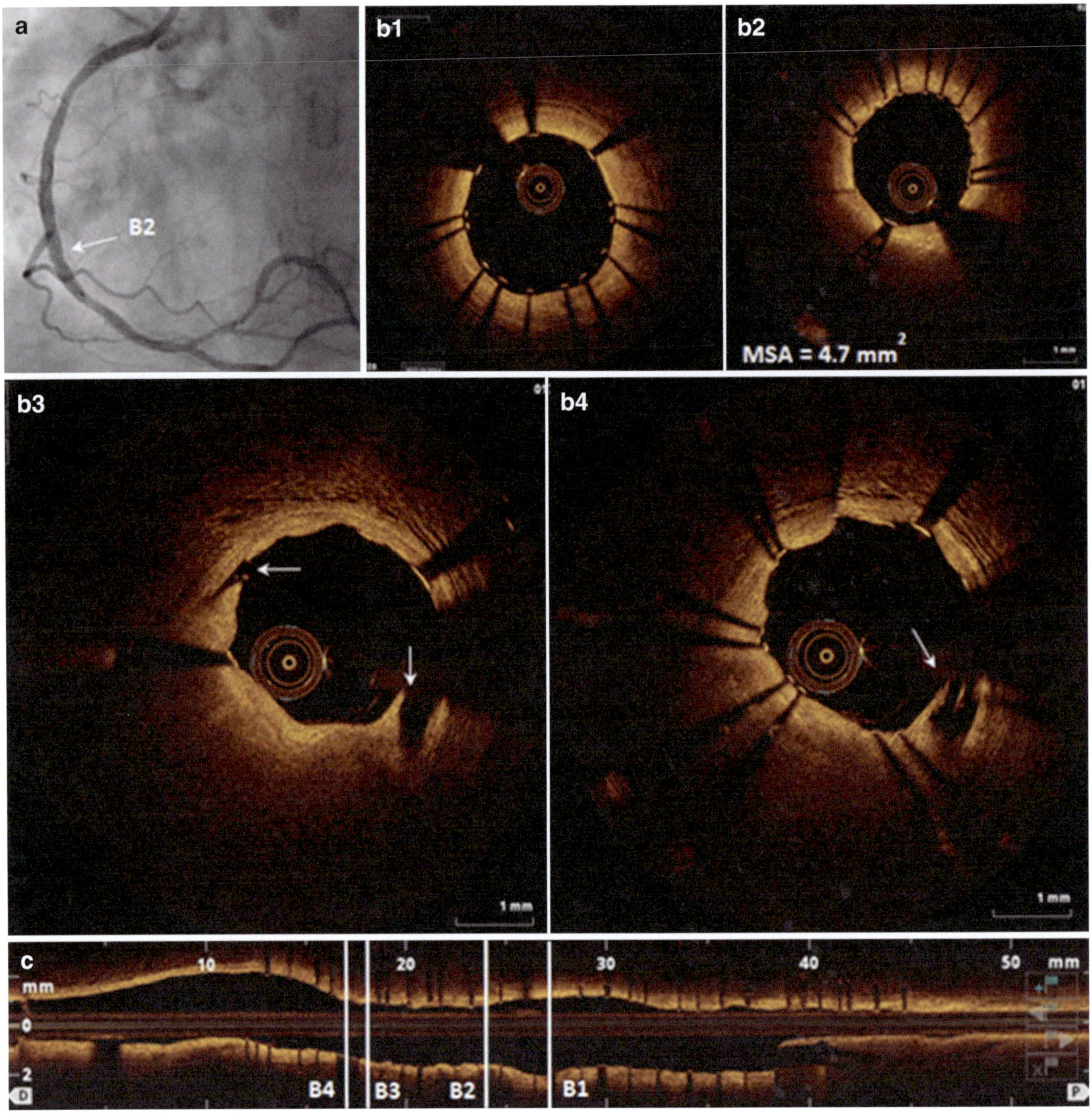

Fig. 4.6 Angiography and OCT after postdilatation. There was no evidence of stent malapposition after dilatation (**b1**, **b2**). In addition to improved stent apposition, OCT showed improved stent expansion after postdilatation with MSA (**b2**). Slightly deeper intima-media in-stent dissections were detected distal to the site of MSA after postdilatation; the dissections were not visible on angiogram (**a**). In conclusion, detection of suboptimal stent expansion by OCT resulted in postdilatation, which led to an increase in MSA and a slightly deeper tissue injury

4.4 Case 3. Stent Underexpansion in a Calcified Bifurcation Lesion (Figs. 4.7, 4.8 and 4.9, Videos 4.7, 4.8 and 4.9)

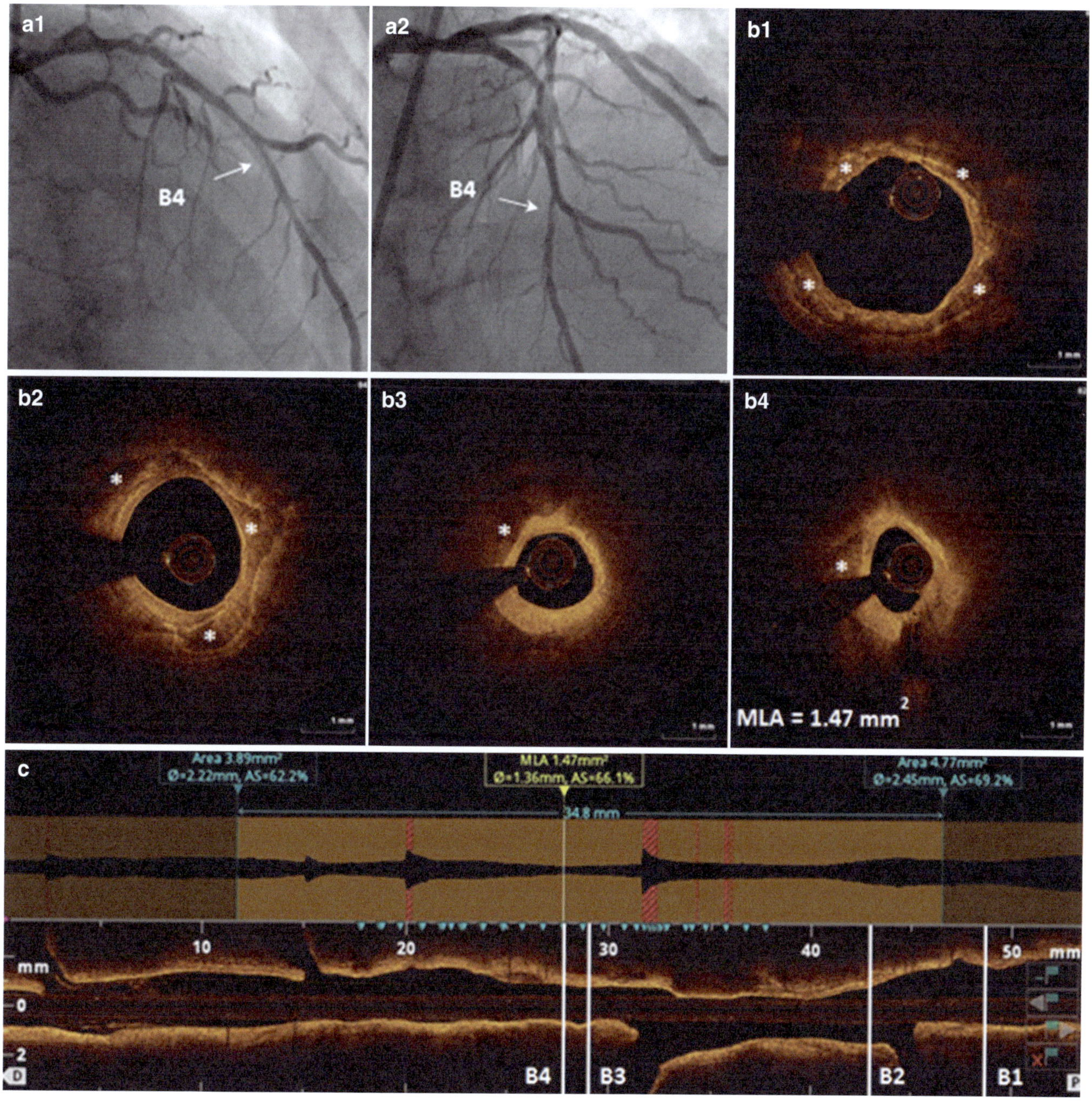

Fig. 4.7 Coronary angiography and OCT imaging before PCI. A 64-year-old male with controlled hypertension, hyperlipidemia, NIDDM, a history of prior MI, and multiple PCI presented for a staged intervention of the LAD. A 70–80% calcified lesion was detected in the mid-LAD by angiography (**a1**, **a2**). OCT pullback confirmed the severity of the disease with MLA of 1.47 mm² and 66% stenosis measured using automatic lumen profile tool (**c**). In addition, OCT detected severe circumferential calcification proximal to the MLA site (**b1**, **b2**, *asterisks*) and moderate (1–2 quadrant) calcified plaques at the site of the MLA (**b3**, **b4**). Based on OCT analysis of calcium distribution, rotational atherectomy (RA) was performed in the mid LAD using 1.75 mm burr at 150,000 rpm followed by placement of a 3/38 mm DES

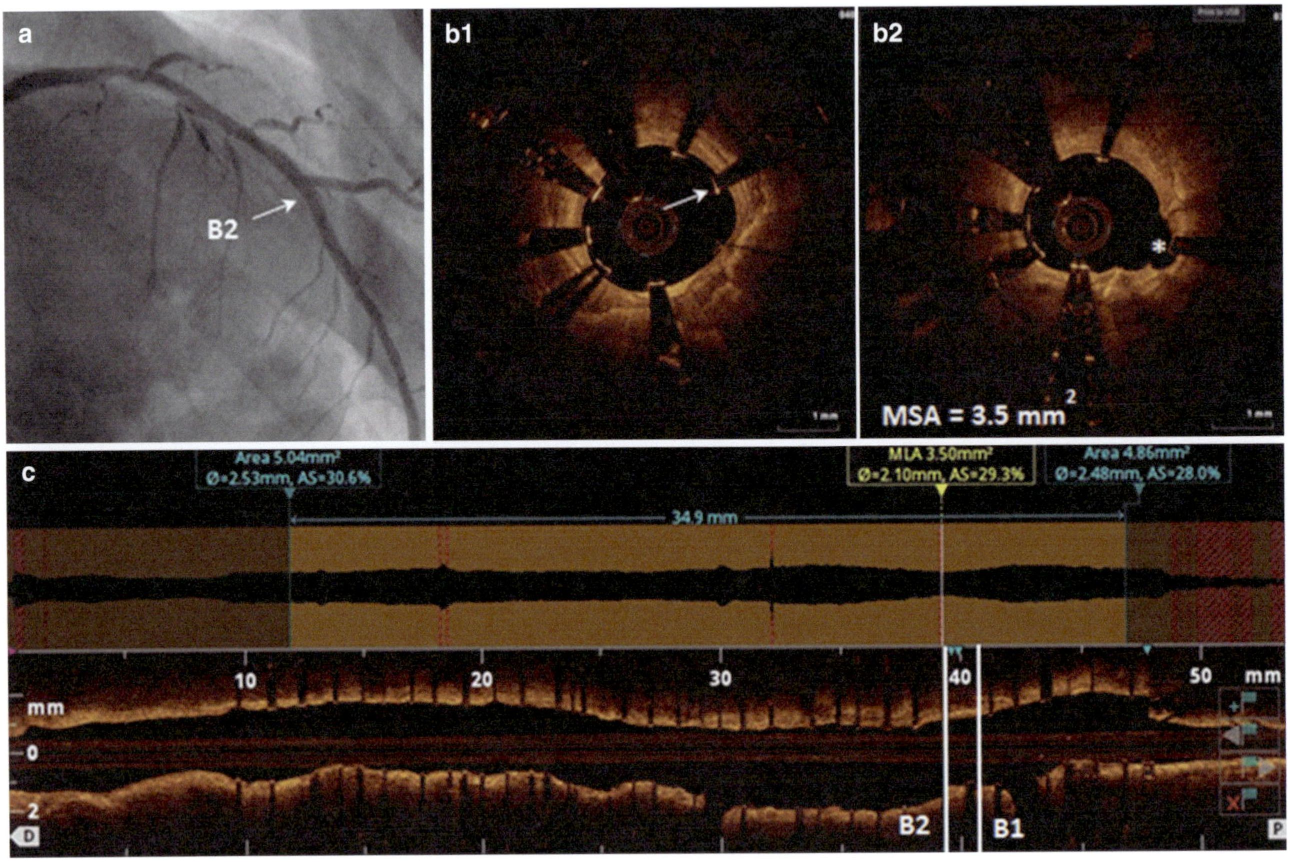

Fig. 4.8 Coronary angiogram (**a**) and OCT after RA and stenting. Post-stent OCT detected few malapposed struts (**b1**) and suboptimal stent expansion at the level of circumferential calcification (**b2**, **c**). While there was OCT evidence of plaque modifications with RA (**b2**, *asterisk*), automatic lumen profile showed a 29% residual stenosis and minimal stent area of 3.5 mm^2 after stenting. Postdilatation was performed with a 3.5/15 mm noncompliant balloon at 20 atm for 10 s

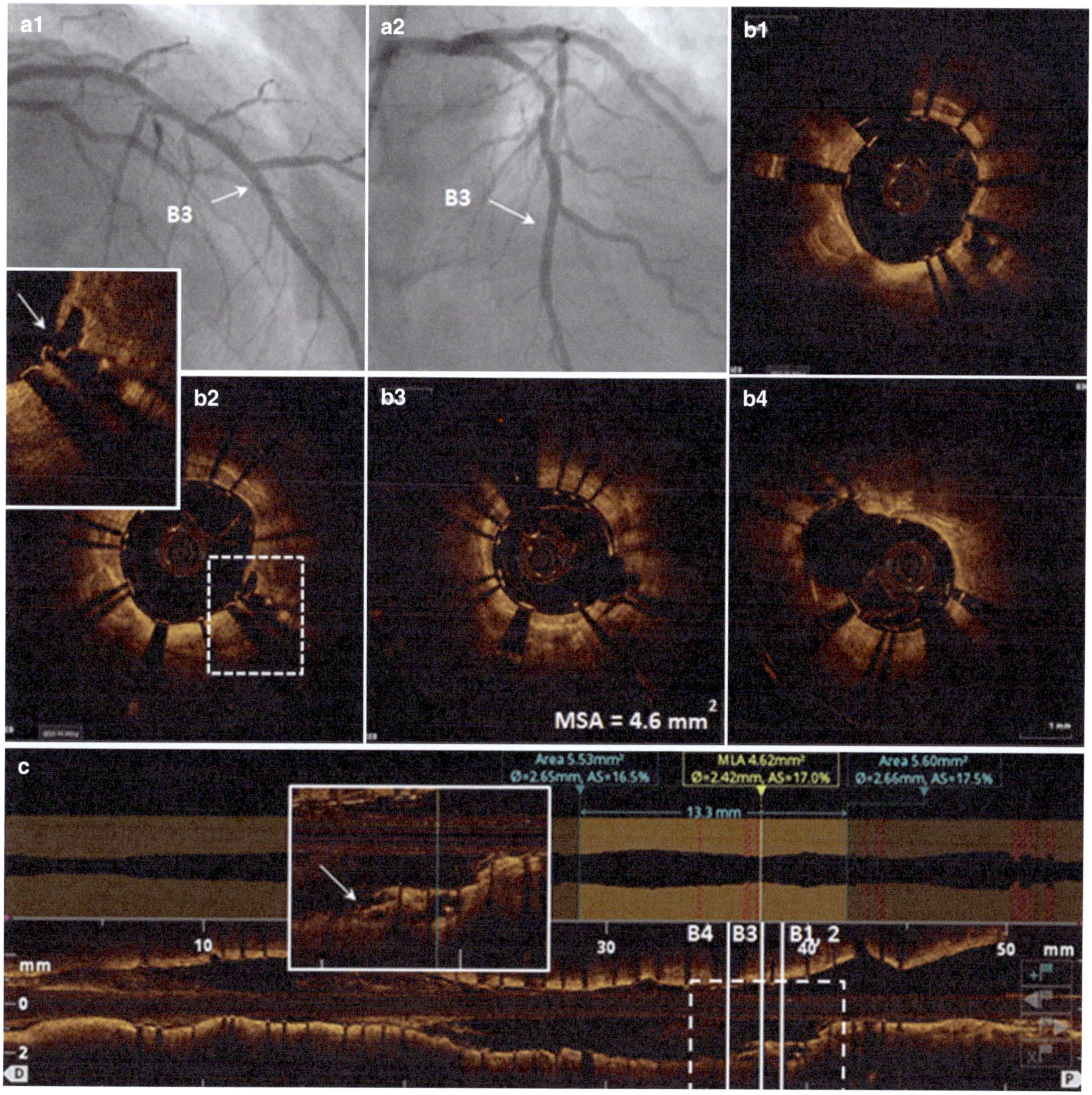

Fig. 4.9 Coronary angiography (**a1, a2**) and OCT imaging after postdilatation. OCT demonstrated improved stent expansion with MSA of 4.6 mm² (**b3**) and resolved malapposition (**b4**). In addition, OCT uncovered more substantial plaque modifications after postdilatation with visible cracks within calcified plaque proximal to MSA at the site of 360° calcification (**b1**, **b2**-inset, and C-inset). In this case, OCT imaging before PCI confirmed the presence of severe calcification and provided guidance for calcium ablation with rotational atherectomy. Post-stent OCT detected stent underexpansion, which was resolved after postdilatation

4.5 Case 4. Acute Stent Thrombosis (Fig. 4.10, Video 4.10)

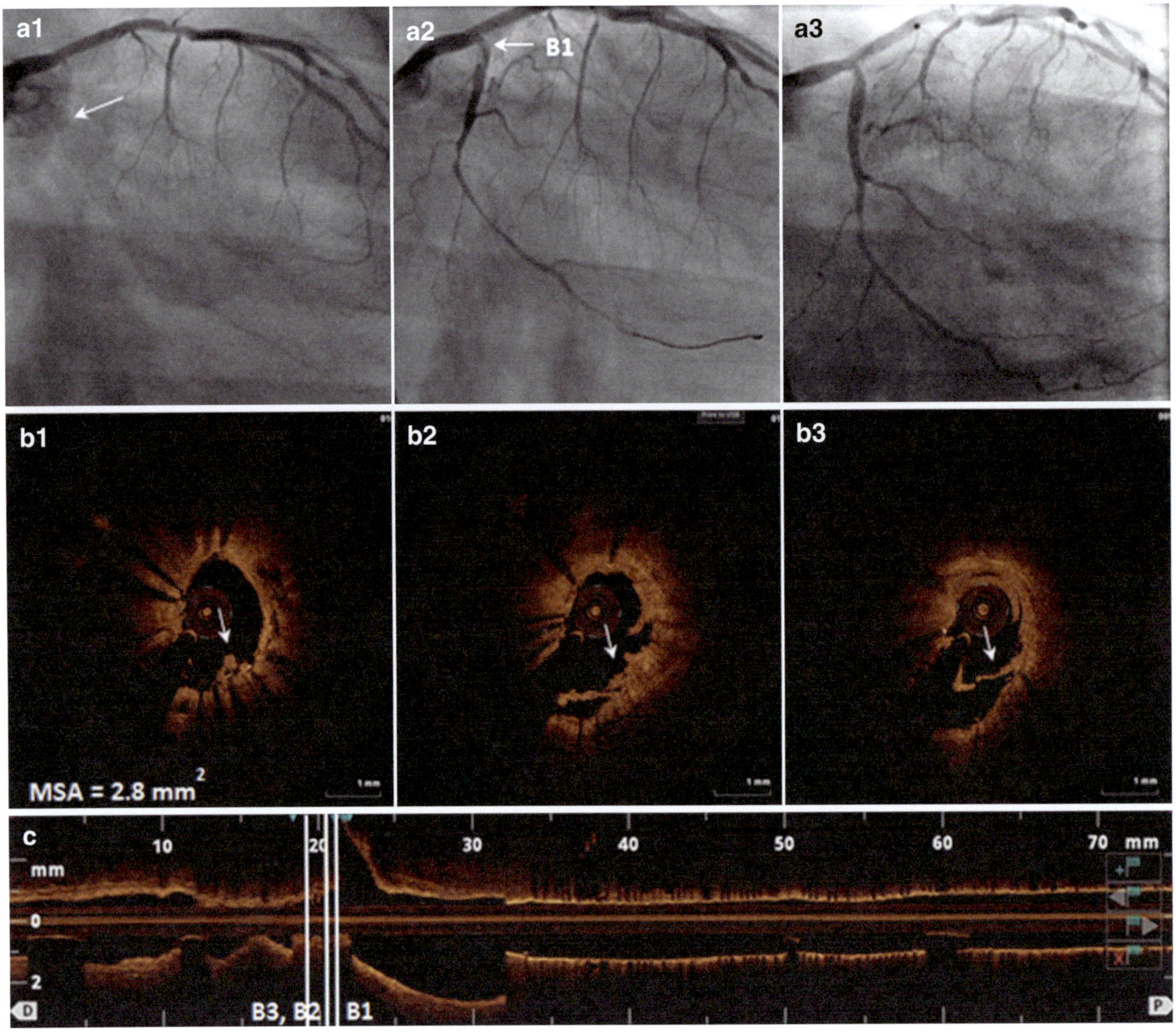

Fig. 4.10 Coronary angiogram and OCT imaging in a patient with acute stent thrombosis. A 49-year-old female with controlled hypertension and hyperlipidemia, uncontrolled DM, multiple prior PCI, and recent NSTEMI had a PCI with a 2.5/12 mm everolimus-eluting stent to the proximal LCX. Thirteen hours after the intervention, the patient developed chest pain and elevated troponin (cTnI 12.6). Coronary angiogram confirmed stent thrombosis resulting in total occlusion of the LCX (**a1**, *arrow*). Coronary angiogram performed after thrombus aspiration and postdilatation with a 2/12 mm noncompliant balloon is shown in A2. OCT imaging of the proximal LCX visualized residual thrombus inside the stent (**b1**–**b3**, *arrow*) and detected stent underexpansion with the minimal stent area 2.8 mm^2 (**b1**). Postdilatation with 2.5/15 and 2.75/12 mm noncompliant balloon at 20 atm led to satisfactory angiographic results (**a3**). In this case, OCT helped uncover stent underexpansion as the main mechanism of acute stent thrombosis and led to a decision to proceed with postdilatation to achieve optimal stent expansion

4.6 Case 5. Subacute Stent Thrombosis (Figs. 4.11 and 4.12, Videos 4.11 and 4.12)

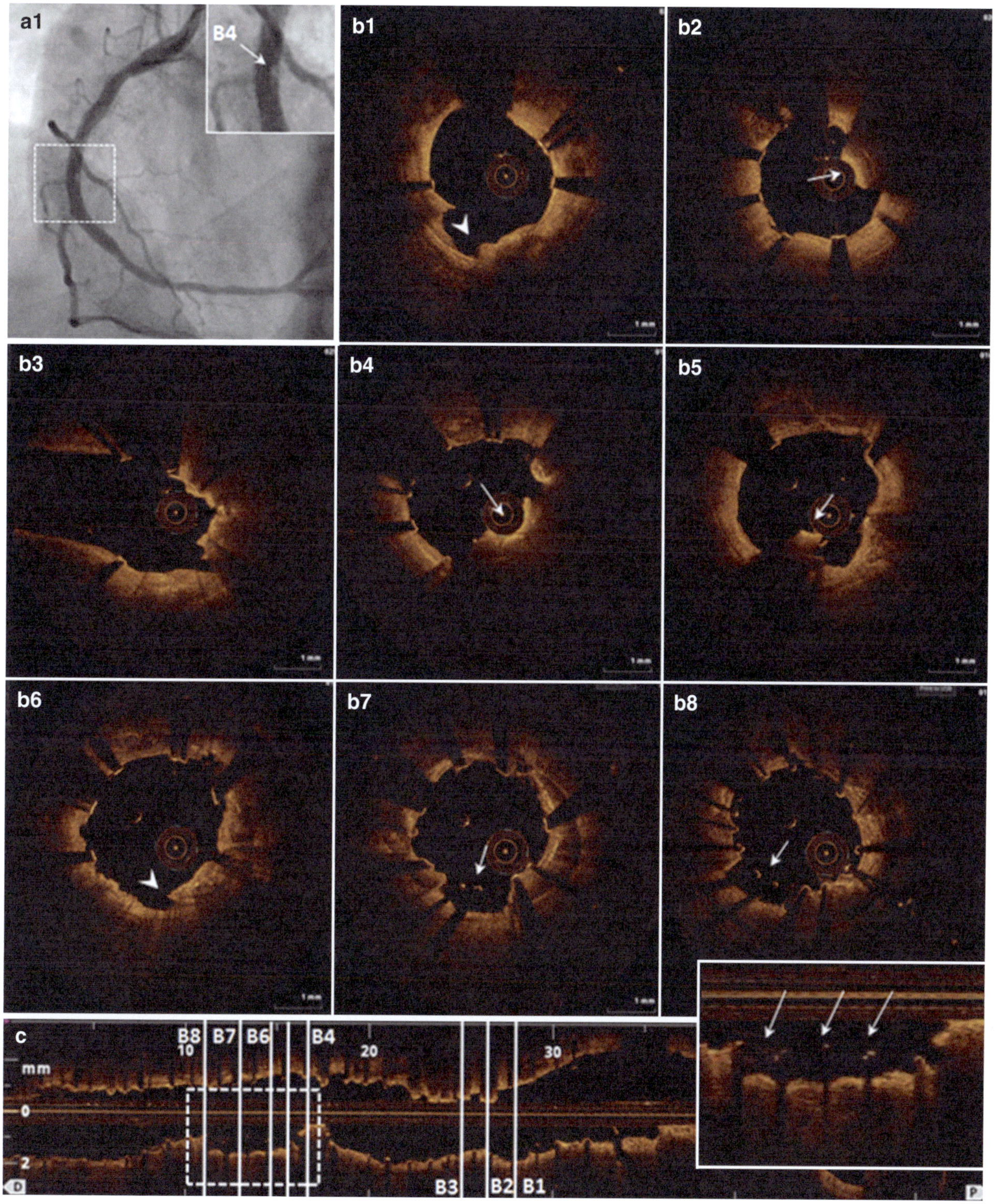

Fig. 4.11 A 59-year-old male with controlled hypertension, NIDDM, and hyperlipidemia was treated for NSTEMI with a 3/32 mm DES to the RCA. Eleven days after the intervention, the patient presented with CCS class IV angina. Coronary angiography revealed a focal thrombotic lesion in the mid portion of the RCA (**a**, inset). OCT imaging confirmed subacute stent thrombosis by visualizing two separate non-occlusive thrombi within the stent (**b2** and **b4**, **b5**, *arrow*). While the large distal thrombus (**b4**, **b5**) was visualized by angiography (**a**, *arrow*), the smaller proximal thrombus (**b2**) was not visible on angiogram. In addition, OCT detected significant stent strut malapposition around heavy calcification with a total longitudinal length of 6 mm (**b7**, **b8**, and C-inset, *arrows*) in-stent dissection (**b6**, *arrowhead*) just distal to the larger thrombus. There was also in-stent dissection and soft plaque protrusion around the proximal thrombus (**b1**, *arrowhead*). Based on the OCT findings, additional stent dilatation was performed

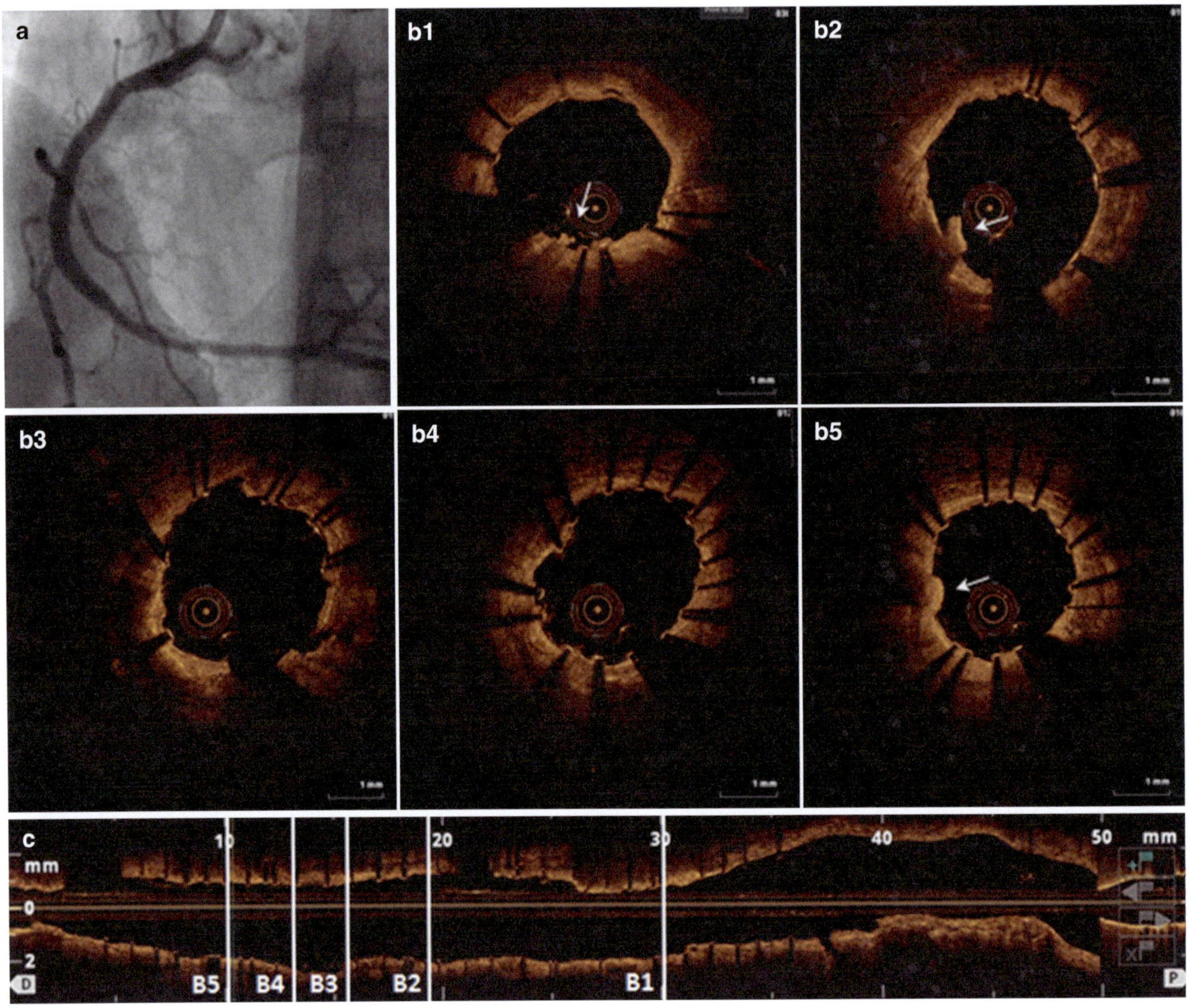

Fig. 4.12 Post PCI angiogram and OCT imaging. Coronary angiogram showed a satisfactory result after stent dilatation with a 3.5/12 mm noncompliant balloon at 20 atm (**a**). OCT imaging further verified significantly improved stent strut apposition around severe calcified plaque (**b3**–**b5**). Small-tissue protrusion (**b5**, *arrow*) and minimal residual thrombotic burden were detected in several OCT frames (**b1**, **b2**, *arrow*). After PCI, patient was switched from clopidogrel to ticagrelor therapy. Based on pre-PCI OCT imaging, stent strut malapposition was suggested as the main mechanism of subacute stent thrombosis in this case. Post-PCI OCT imaging verified adequate stent apposition after additional stent dilatation

4.7 Case 6. Another Case of Subacute Stent Thrombosis (Figs. 4.13 and 4.14, Videos 4.13 and 4.14)

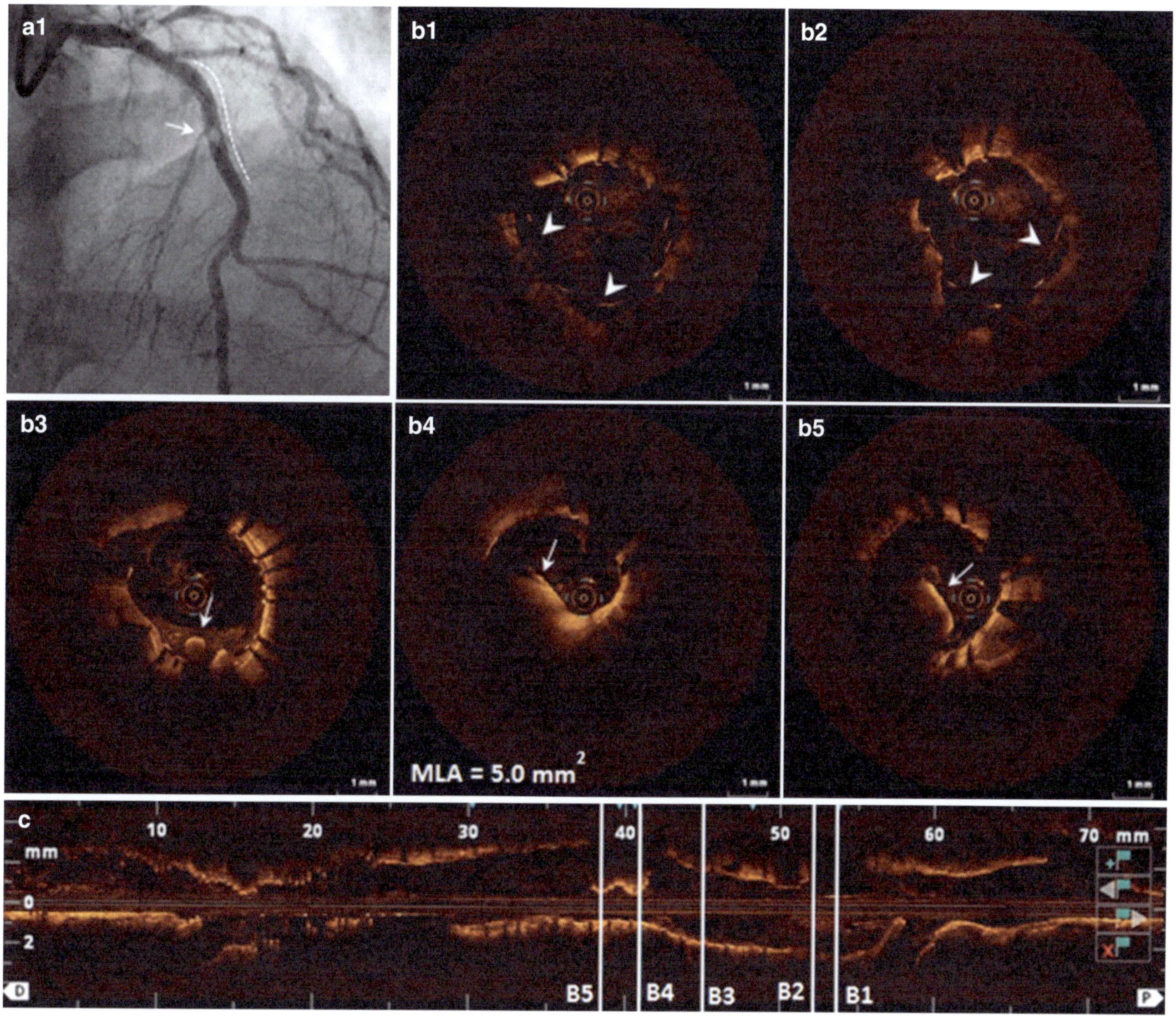

Fig. 4.13 A 38-year-old male with a history of hypertension, hyperlipidemia, failed renal transplant, peritoneal dialysis, Plavix non-responder with P2Y12 Reaction Units (PRU) of 420 had a PCI with rotational atherectomy and a 3.5/33 mm DES implantation in the mid LAD. Twenty-eight days after the intervention, the patient presented with chest pain on minimal exertion and at rest while being on dual antiplatelet therapy. Coronary angiography showed thrombus formation (**a1**, *arrow*) inside the LAD stent (**a1**, *dotted line*). OCT imaging confirmed stent thrombosis demonstrating a large red thrombus in the center of the stent (**b4**, **b5**, *arrow*) at the minimal lumen area site (**b4**) and a smaller thrombus proximal to the MLA (**b3**, *arrow*). Although stent area assessment was not possible in some frames due to the overlying thrombus, stent expansion was characterized as adequate. Stent malapposition was detected at the proximal edge of the stent (**b1**, **b2**, *arrowhead*)

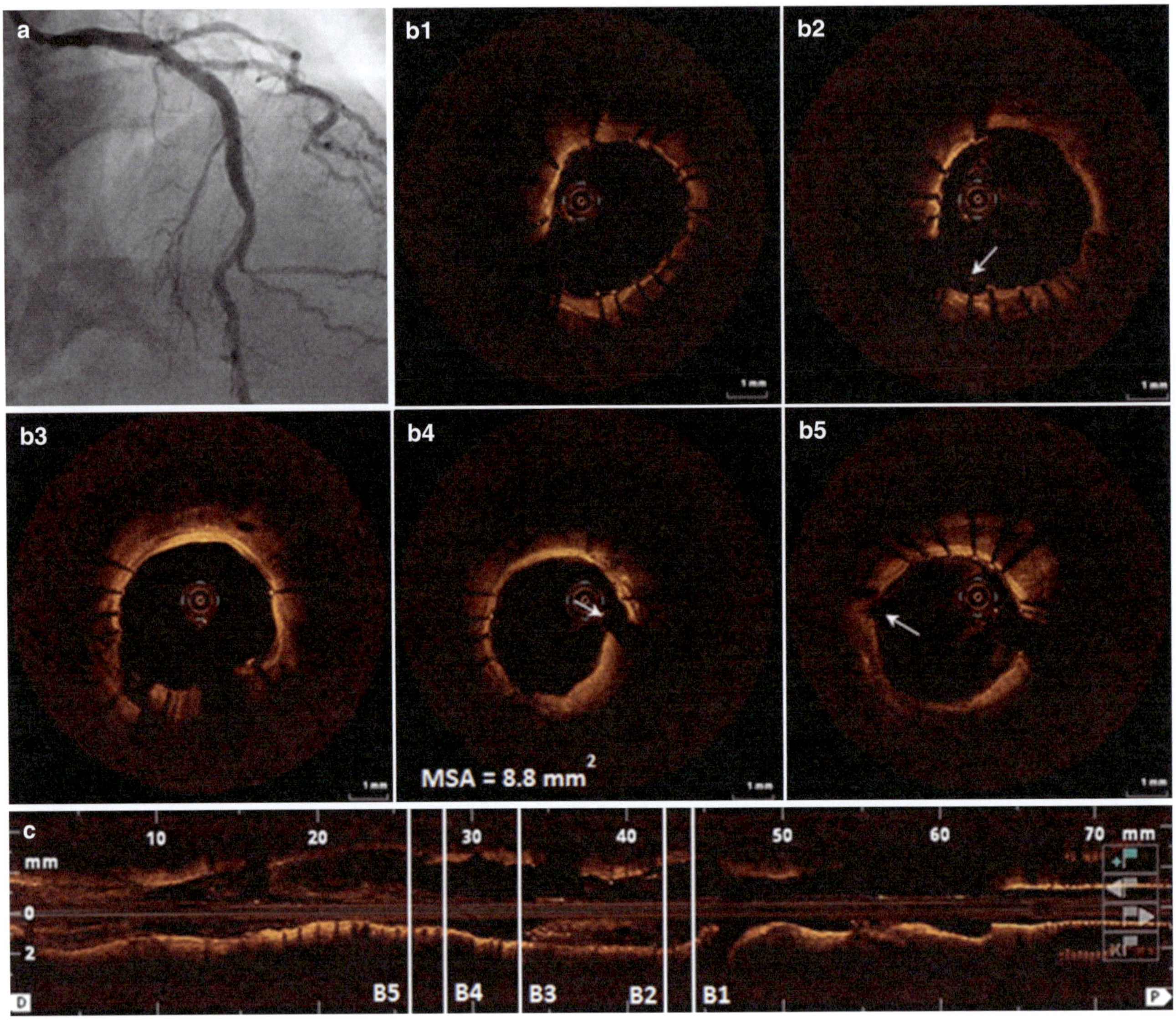

Fig. 4.14 Final post-PCI angiogram and OCT. Thrombectomy and cutting balloon angioplasty were successful in achieving a satisfactory angiographic result (**a**). OCT demonstrated improved stent expansion (**b4**) and apposition at the proximal edge of the stent (**b1**, **b2**) with few malapposed struts still present in several frames (**b2**, *arrow*). There was no residual thrombus remaining in the vessel; small intimal dissections, either previously covered by thrombus or newly formed as a result of postdilatation, were detected in the center of the stent (**b4**, **b5**, *arrow*). Patient was switched from clopidogrel to ticagrelor therapy

4.8 Case 7. Establishing a Track (Fig. 4.15)

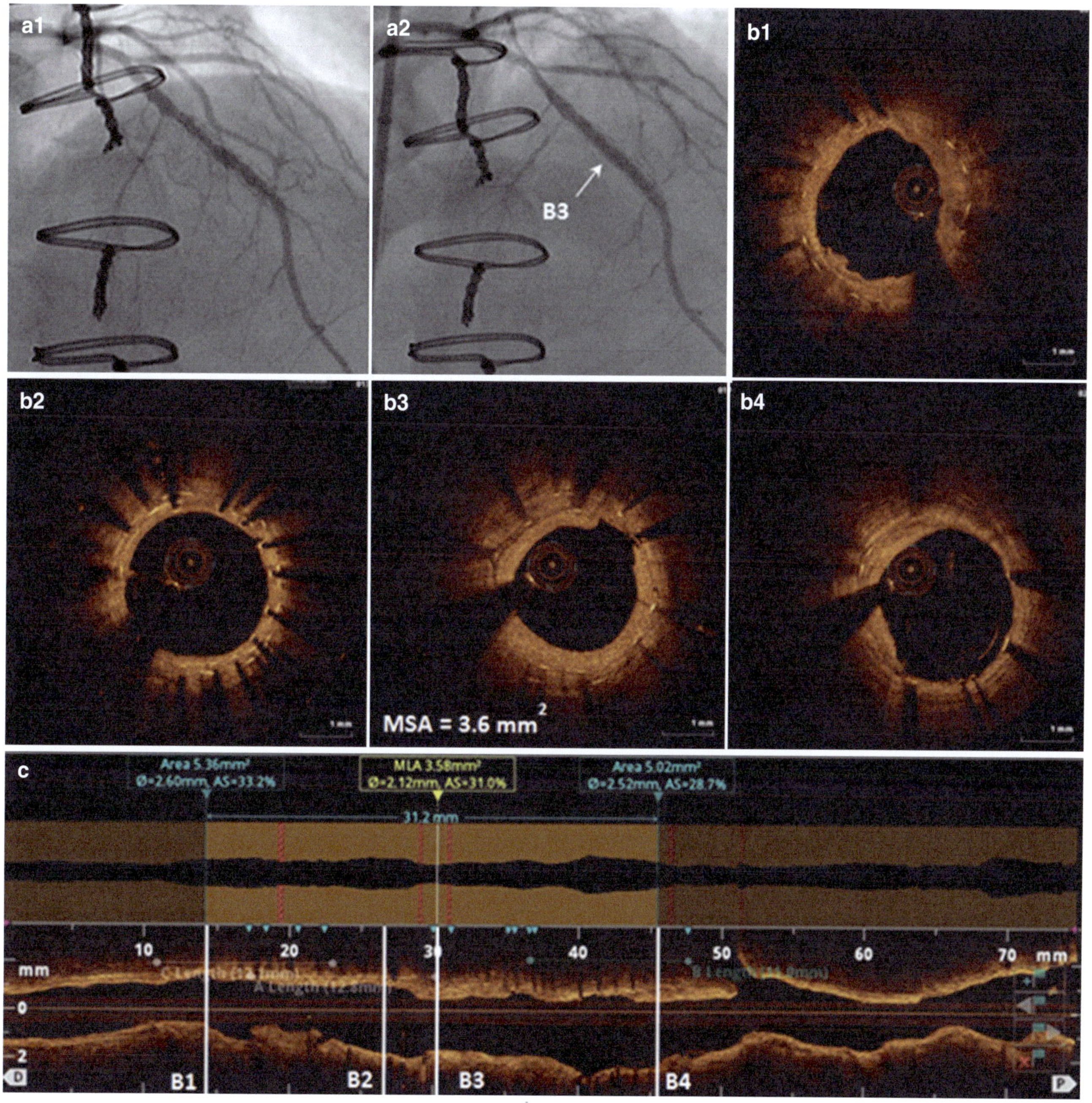

Fig. 4.15 Coronary angiography and OCT images of a 73-year-old male with a history of multiple PCIs and coronary artery bypass surgery (CABG), who presented with CCS Class II angina and exertional shortness of breath. SPECT MPI suggested moderate basal anteroseptal ischemia. CABG with LIMA to the mid-LAD grafting was performed 8 years prior, and the last documented PCI was a 2.75/12 mm DES to the mid-LAD 4 years after the surgery. Coronary angiography showed a 70–80% in-stent restenosis lesion in the mid-LAD and a total occlusion of the graft (**a1**). LAD lesion was treated with rotational atherectomy using 1.75 mm burr at 150,000 rpm for 80 s followed by high-pressure inflation with noncompliant balloon resulting in procedural success demonstrated by angiography (**a2**) and OCT imaging (**b1**–**b4**, **c**). In addition to the documented DES stent, OCT uncovered two previously deployed stents in the same area. Three stent layers (**b2**) were detected distal to the MLA site (**b3**). Two stent layers were visualized at the minimal lumen area site (**b3**) and in the 10-mm adjacent proximal segment. One stent layer was detected at the proximal (**b4**) and distal site of the lesion (**b1**). Based on OCT findings, the operator proceeded with brachytherapy as the preferred treatment for the recurrent restenosis of the LAD. In the present case, OCT findings on the number and distribution of previously implanted stents helped select vascular brachytherapy without repeat stenting as treatment strategy

4.9 Case 8. Establishing a Track in Rocky Terrain (Fig. 4.16, Video 4.15)

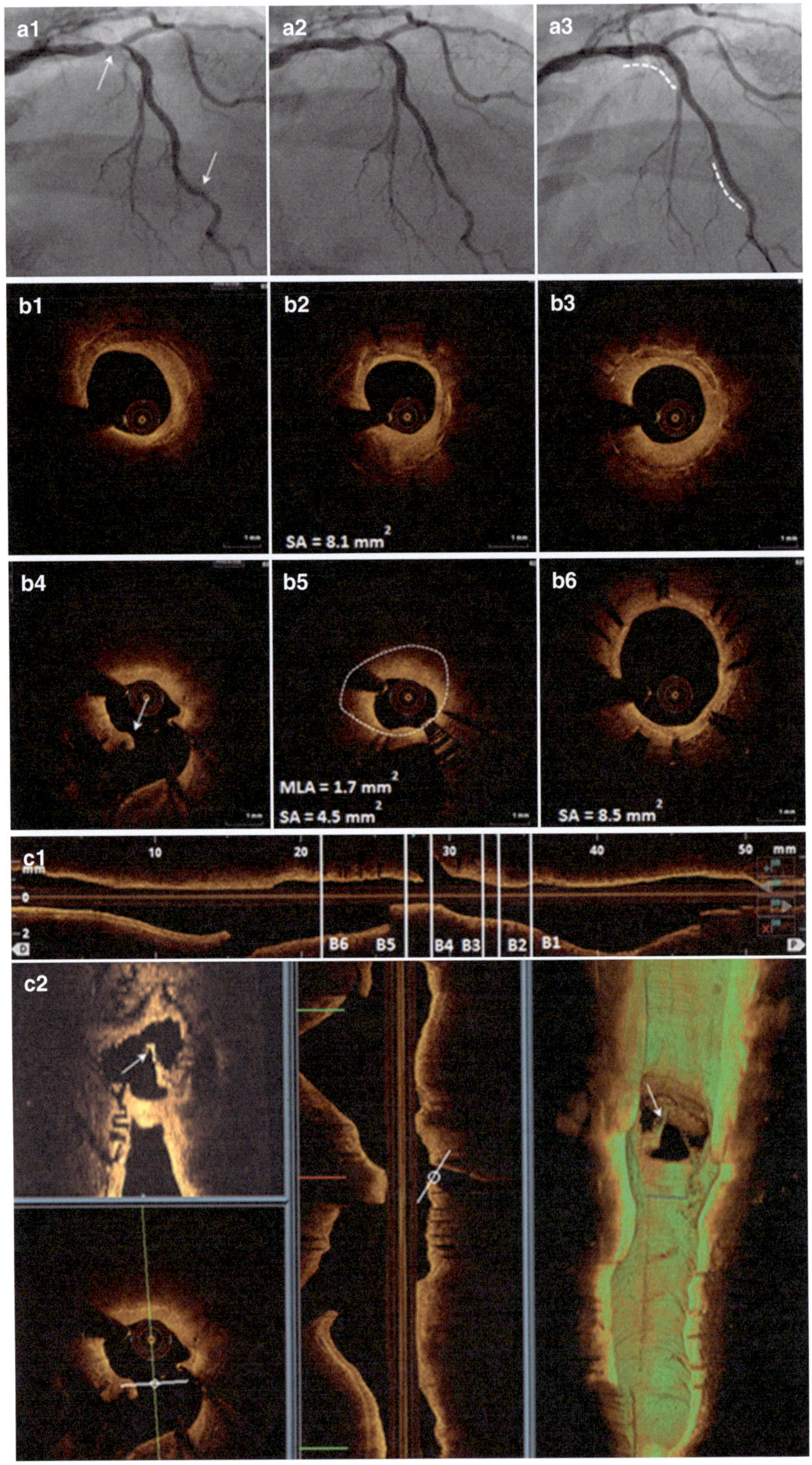

Fig. 4.16 Angiography, two- and three-dimensional OCT imaging of a 62-year-old male with a history of controlled hypertension, IDDM, and multiple PCIs, who was admitted for intervention for LAD-D1 bifurcation lesion. Coronary angiography revealed a 70–80% LAD-D1 ISR lesion and 80–90% severe calcified lesion in the mid-LAD. OCT pullback of the proximal LAD uncovered a focal eccentric in-stent restenosis (**b2**–**b5**) lesion. Proximal to the bifurcation, the lesion was characterized by the presence of circumferential calcification proximal to the stent edge (**b1**) and inside the stent (**b2**, **b3**), mostly lipid-laden plaque around MLA (**b5**) and bifurcation (**b4**). Assessment of stent area (SA) at the proximal reference (**b2**), minimal area (**b5**), and distal reference site (**b6**) demonstrated a 54% stent expansion. Furthermore, OCT showed that angiographic "stent jailing" was due to the neointimal tissue covering stent struts overlying the side branch (**b4**, **c2**, *arrow*) leading to significant reduction of the side branch ostium area. Rotational atherectomy with 1.75 mm burr size at 150,000 rpm was used to ablate the calcified intrastent tissue and calcification in mid-LAD lesion (**a2**) allowing subsequent vessel dilatation. A cutting balloon angioplasty was performed in the side branch followed by the final kissing balloon inflation (KBI) using noncompliant balloons. 3.5/23 and 2.5/23 mm stents were successfully implanted in the proximal and mid-LAD (**a3**)

4.10 Case 9. Orbital Atherectomy for In-Stent Restenosis Lesion (Fig. 4.17, Videos 4.16 and 4.17)

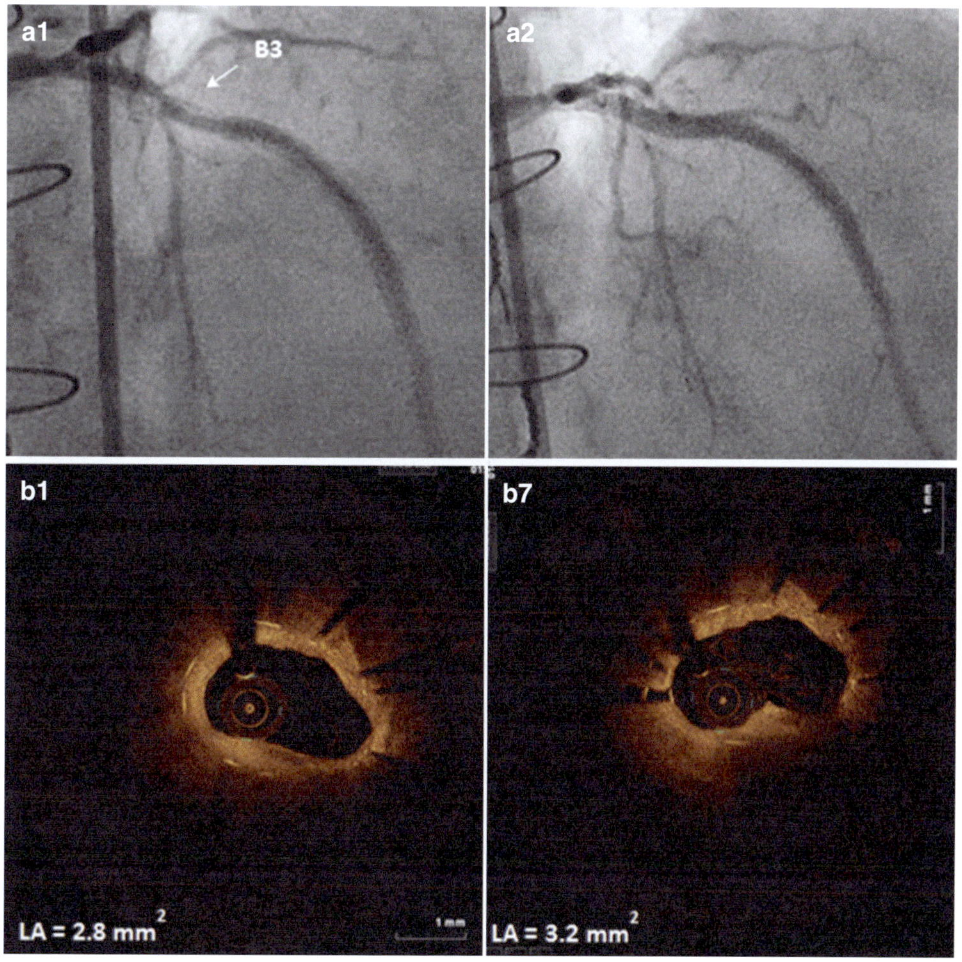

Fig. 4.17 (**a–c**) A 67-year-old female with controlled hypertension, IDDM, hyperlipidemia, and a history of prior MI, CABG, and multiple PCIs presented with CCS Class III angina. The most recent PCI was a 3/38 mm DES implantation in the mid-LAD 6 months earlier. Abnormal MPI demonstrated ischemia involving anterior wall. Angiography showed a 70–80% in-stent restenosis in the proximal and mid-LAD (**a1**). OCT visualized an ISR lesion with minimal lumen area of 1.9 mm^2 and mostly homogeneous fibrotic intrastent tissue inside one layer of stent (**b1–b5**, **c1**). A large calcified plaque was detected outside the stent (**b2**, **b3**, **b5**, *asterisk*). Two stent layers with a lower amount of intimal hyperplasia were detected distal the MLA segment (**b6**). Orbital atherectomy (OA) was performed in the proximal and mid-LAD using a 1.25 burr at 80,000 rpm. Post-atherectomy OCT imaging visualized significant plaque modifications with irregular lumen surface within the MLA site (**b7–b11**); minimal lumen area increased from 1.9 to 2.5 mm^2, resulting in an acute lumen gain of 24%. **b7–b12**, Cross-sectional frames after OA corresponding to the pre-atherectomy images shown in panels **b1–b6**. A 3.5/18 mm DES was implanted in the mid-LAD with adequate final stent expansion assessed by angiography (**a2**). Initial assessment of intrastent plaque morphology and distribution by OCT was used to guide plaque ablation by orbital atherectomy. Post-atherectomy OCT allowed to evaluate the extent of plaque modifications and select stenting as preferred treatment strategy in this case

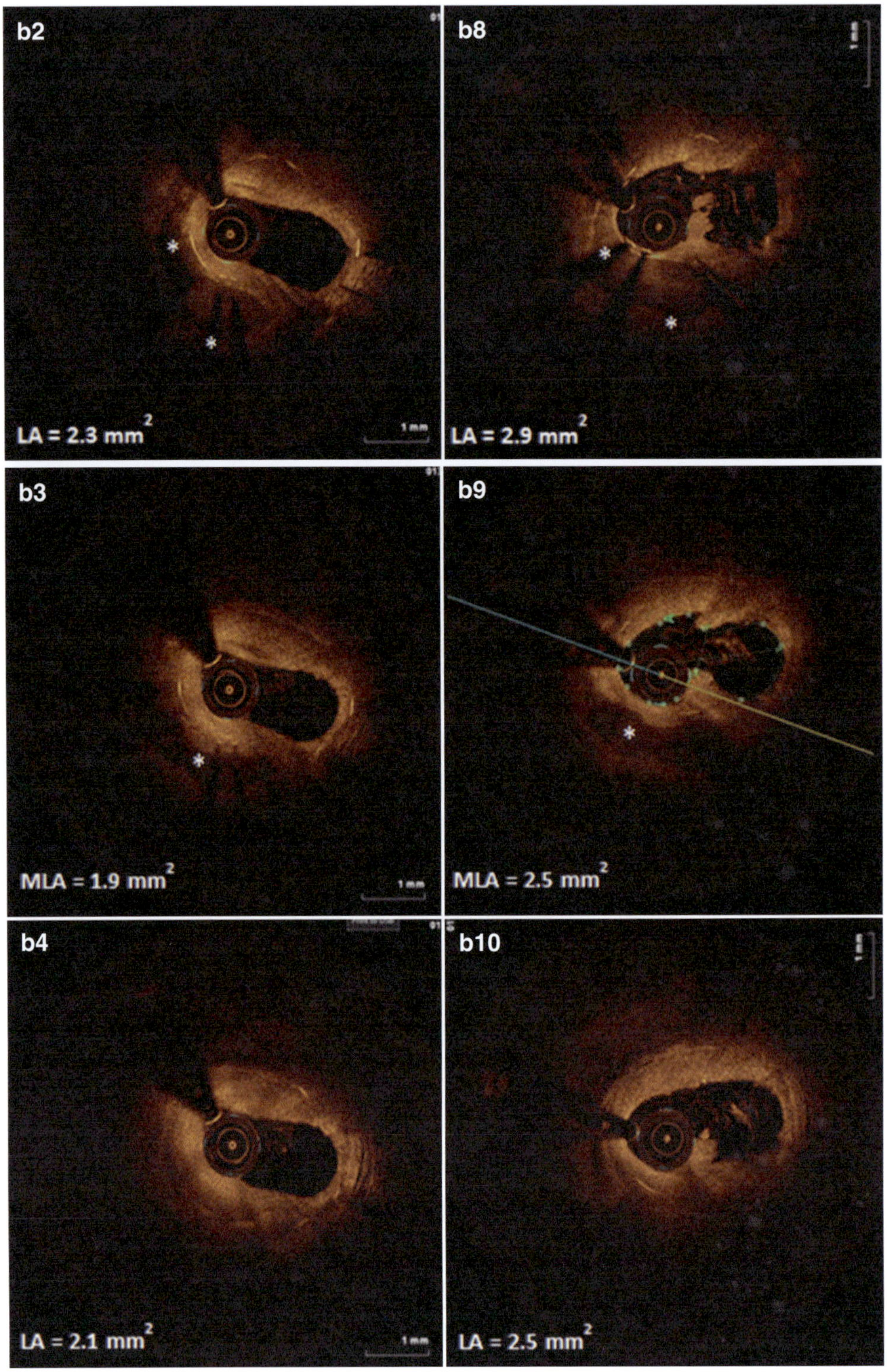

Fig. 4.17 (continued)

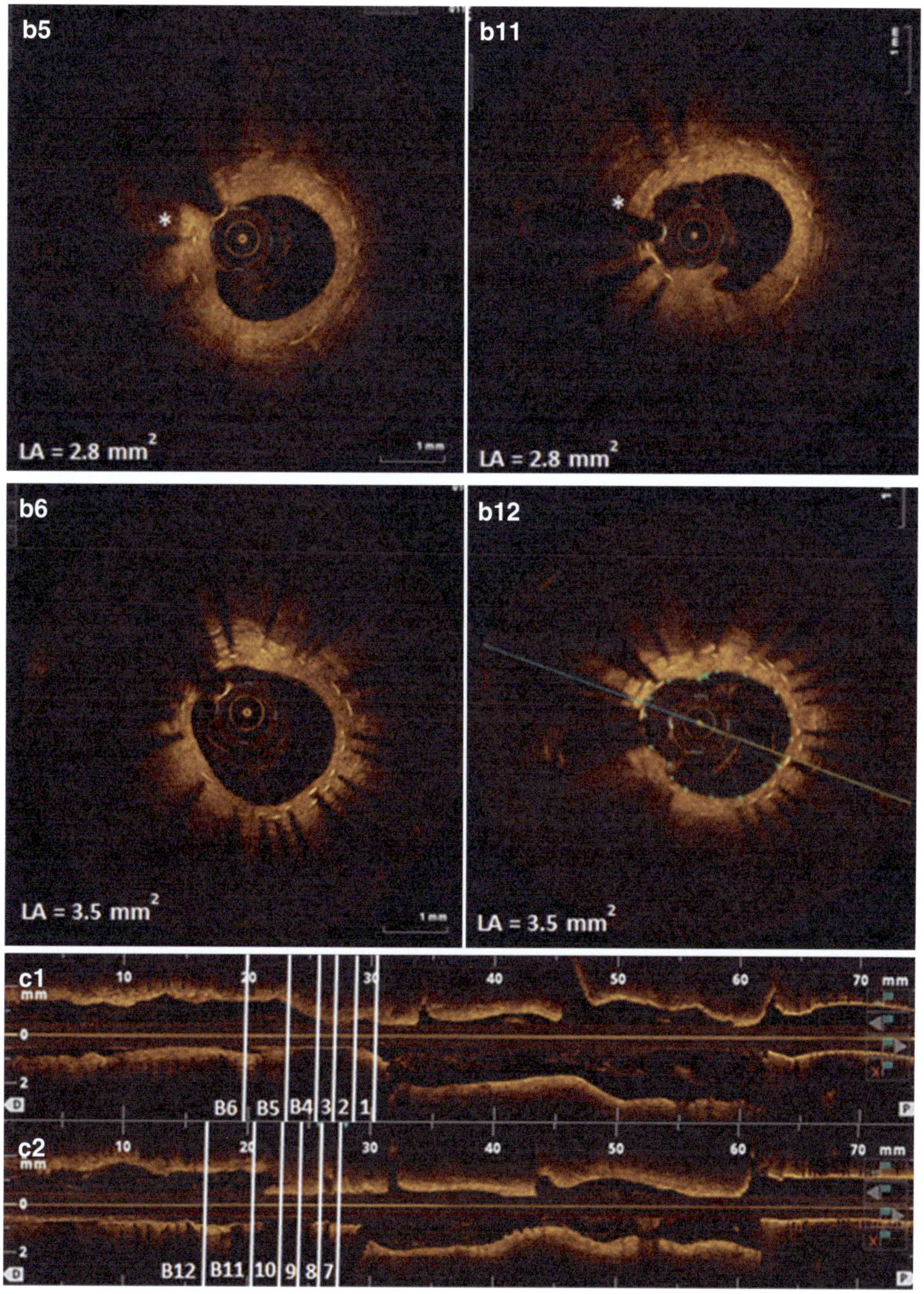

Fig. 4.17 (continued)

4.11 Case 10. Cutting Balloon Angioplasty for In-Stent Restenosis (Figs. 4.18 and 4.19, Videos 4.18 and 4.19)

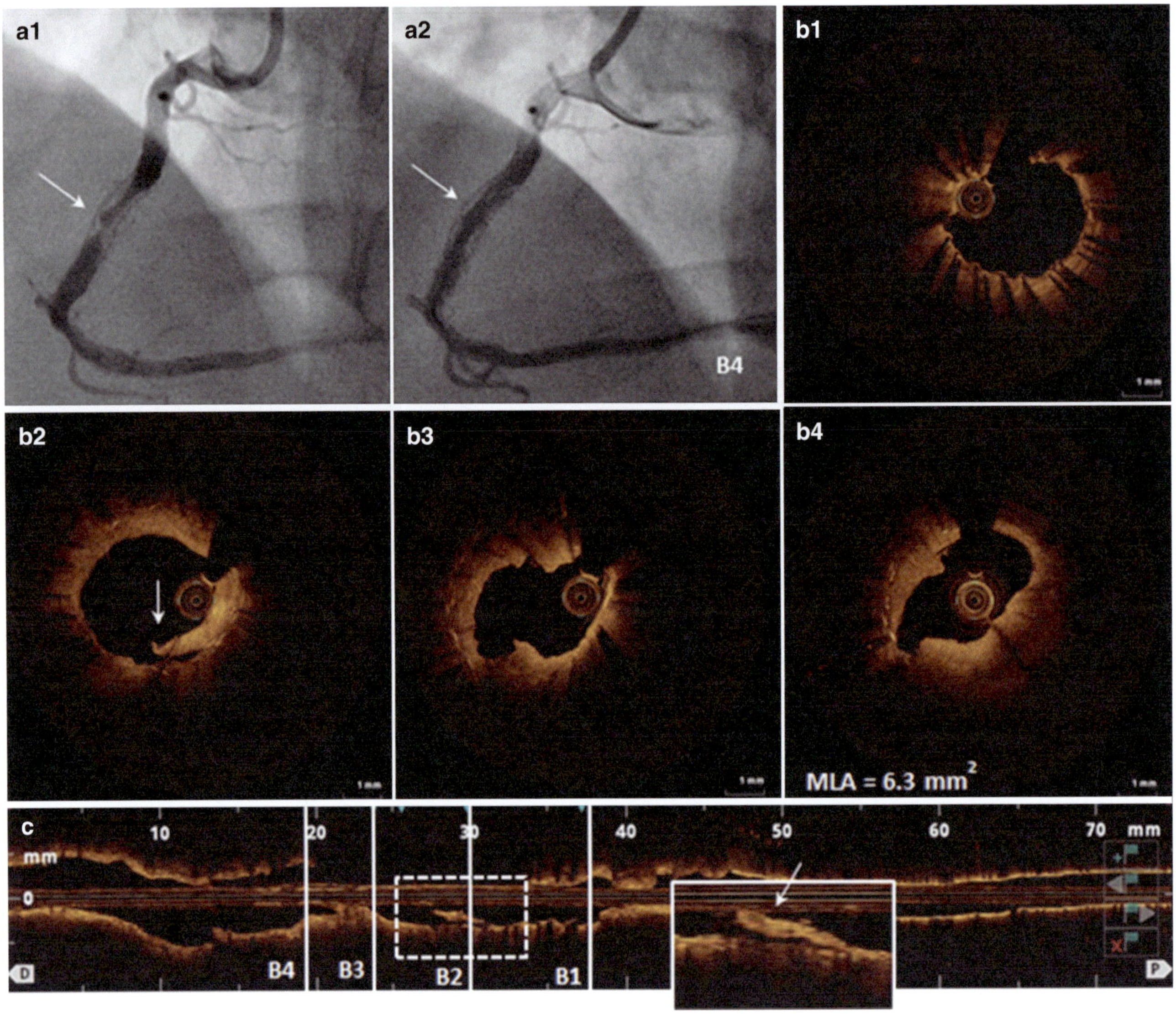

Fig. 4.18 Coronary angiography and OCT before stenting. A 57-year-old male with hyperlipidemia, controlled hypertension, NIDDM, and multiple previous PCI presented with CCS class IV angina. Last intervention was performed 9 months earlier with a DES implanted in the RCA. Coronary angiogram demonstrated a 90–95% diffuse in-stent restenosis of the stent (**a1**, *arrow*). The ISR lesion was treated with a cutting balloon (CB) (4/6 mm Flextome at 12 atm) (**a2**). OCT pullback performed CB angioplasty demonstrated a thin neointimal layer at the proximal (**b1**) and distal stent edges, irregular lumen surface with several intimal fissures and flaps (**b2**–**b4**), including a long intimal flap visible in OCT longitudinal view (**c**-inset, *arrow*). Minimal lumen area was 6.3 mm^2 (**b4**) suggesting effective plaque scoring

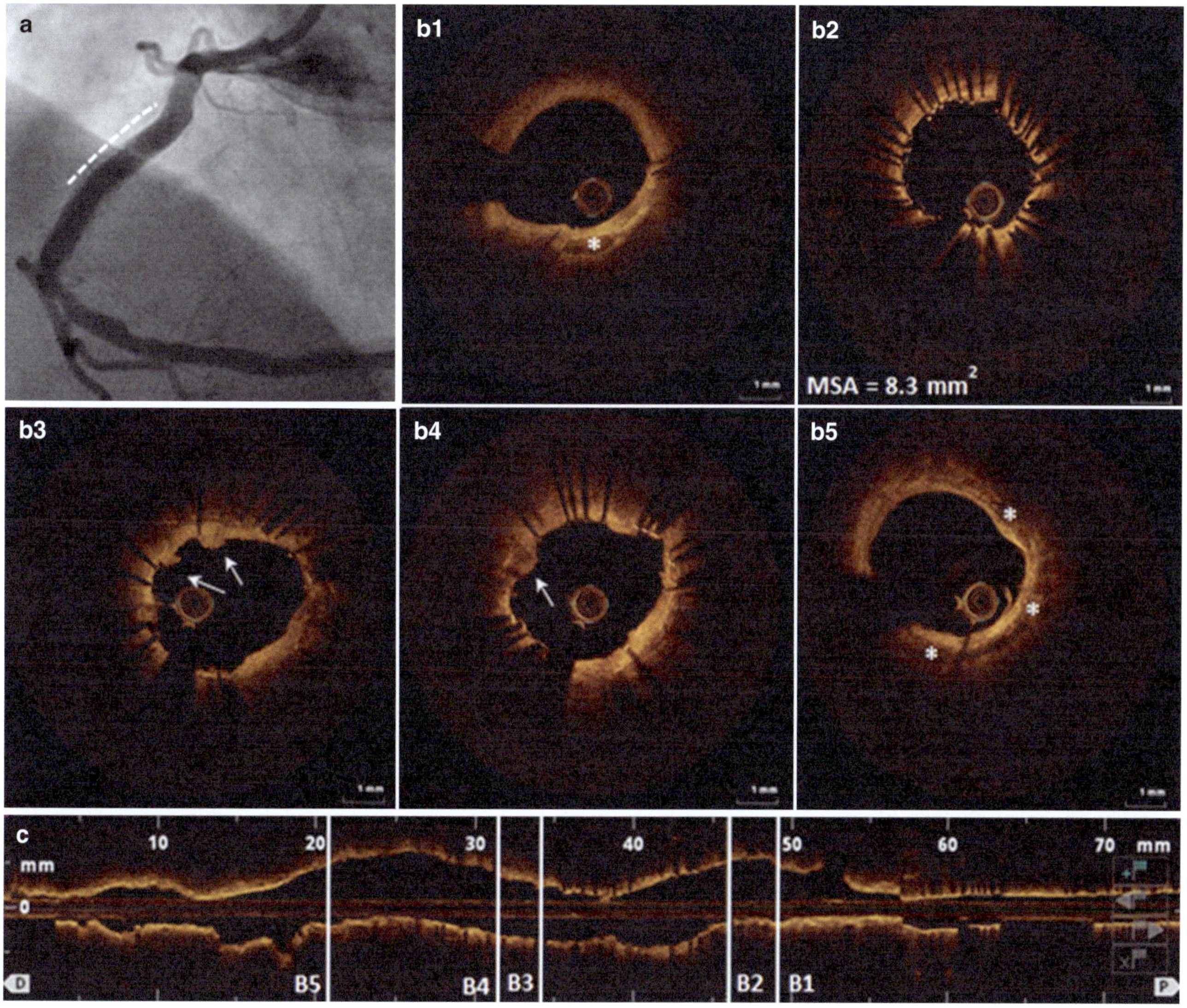

Fig. 4.19 Angiogram and OCT imaging after stenting. Based on the pre-procedural evaluation of lesion morphology and CB effects including a large intimal flap, the operator decided to deploy an additional DES (**a**, *dotted line*). OCT pullback after stent placement confirmed good expansion and apposition of the new stent (**b2–b4**), demonstrated small tissue protrusions (**b3**, **b4**, *arrows*) and didn't detect either distal or proximal stent edge dissection in the presence of calcification (**b1**, **b5**, *asterisks*). OCT imaging after CB was used to analyze the effects of cutting balloon angioplasty and led to a decision to add another stent, based on OCT detection of a large intimal flap after cutting balloon. Post-PCI OCT imaging was used to verify new stent expansion and apposition

4.12 Case 11. In-Stent Restenosis with Chronic Total Occlusion (Figs. 4.20 and 4.21, Videos 4.20 and 4.21)

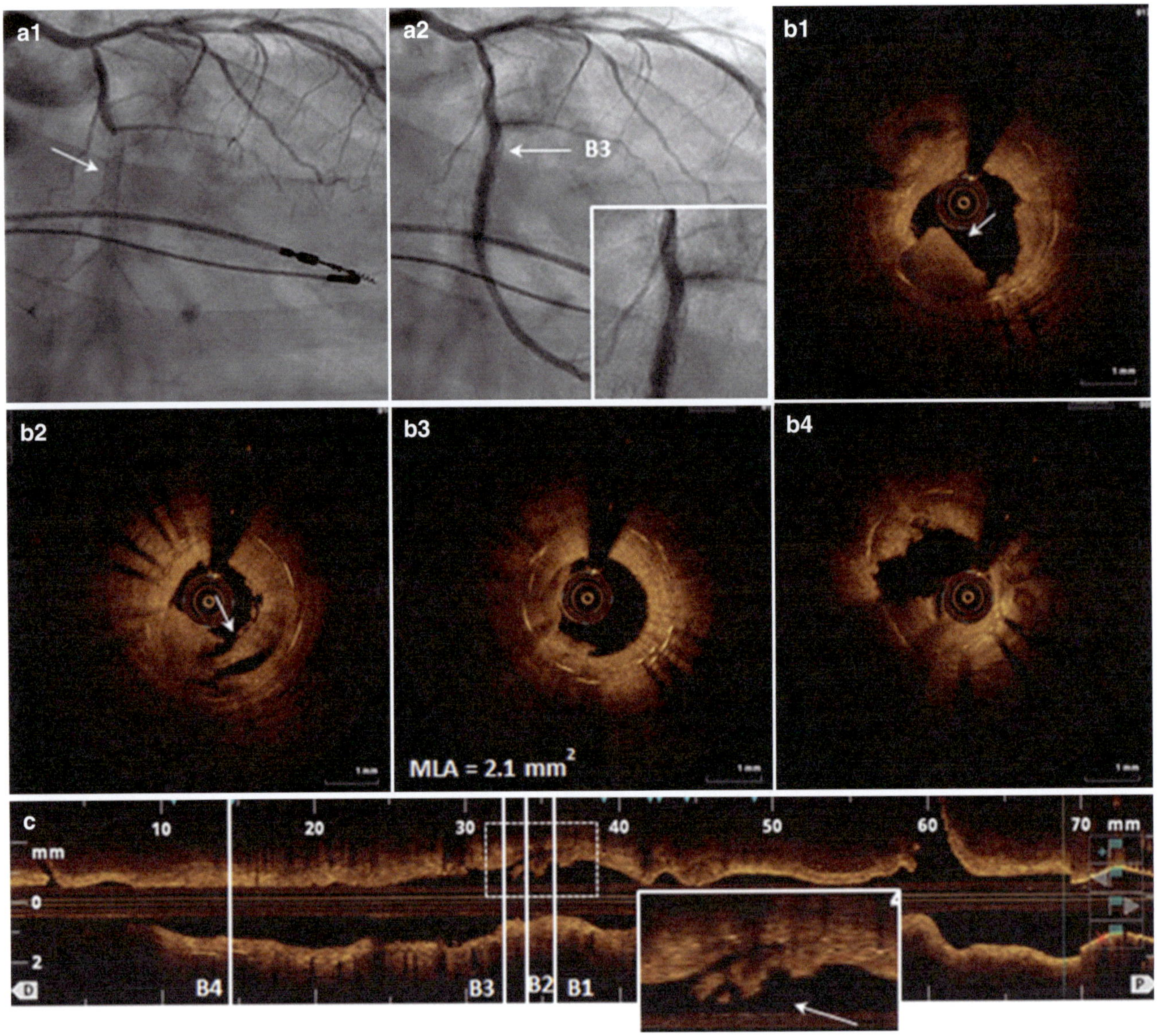

Fig. 4.20 An 81-year-old male with controlled hyperlipidemia, hypertension, and IDDM, prior history of MI, and multiple PCI presented with chest pain, dyspnea on minimal exertion, and positive stress ECG test. Coronary angiography showed in-stent chronic total occlusion (CTO) of the distal LCX (**a1**, *arrow*) filling from bridge collaterals. CTO was crossed using Miracle Bros 3 guidewire (**a2**). OCT pullback visualized significant intimal thickening with an MLA of 2.1 mm^2 (**b3**) and irregular lumen surface with large intimal flaps (**b1**, **b2**, **c**-inset, *arrow*). There was no evidence of calcification detected within the CTO segment. Based on the imaging findings, the lesion was treated with an additional stent

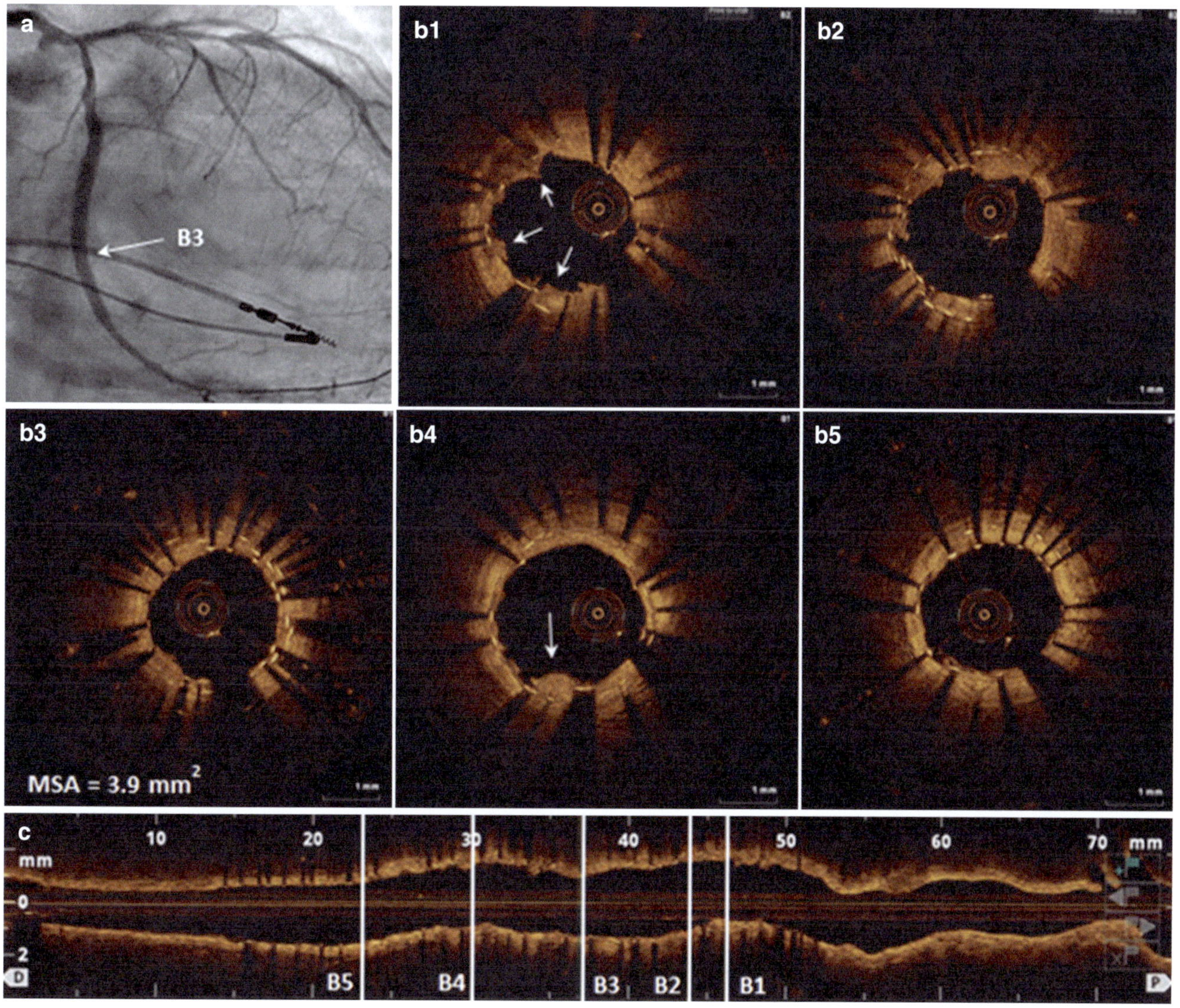

Fig. 4.21 Post-stent angiogram and OCT. An everolimus-eluting 3/38 mm stent was successfully deployed in the LCX (**a**). OCT imaging confirmed good stent expansion and apposition (**b3**) with small tissue protrusions visualized in several OCT frames (**b1**, **b4**, *arrows*)

References

1. Sonoda S, Morino Y, Ako J, Terashima M, Hassan AH, Bonneau HN, et al. Impact of final stent dimensions on long-term results following sirolimus-eluting stent implantation: serial intravascular ultrasound analysis from the sirius trial. J Am Coll Cardiol. 2004;43:1959–63.
2. Doi H, Maehara A, Mintz GS, Yu A, Wang H, Mandinov L, et al. Impact of post-intervention minimal stent area on 9-month follow-up patency of paclitaxel-eluting stents: an integrated intravascular ultrasound analysis from the TAXUS IV, V, and VI and TAXUS ATLAS Workhorse, Long Lesion, and Direct Stent Trials. JACC Cardiovasc Interv. 2009;2:1269–75.
3. Elgendy IY, Mahmoud AN, Elgendy AY, Bavry AA. Outcomes with intravascular ultrasound-guided stent implantation: a meta-analysis of randomized trials in the era of drug-eluting stents. Circ Cardiovasc Interv. 2016;9:e003700.
4. Maehara A, Ben-Yehuda O, Ali Z, Wijns W, Bezerra HG, Shite J, et al. Comparison of stent expansion guided by optical coherence tomography versus intravascular ultrasound: the ILUMIEN II study (observational study of optical coherence tomography [OCT] in patients undergoing fractional flow reserve [ffr] and percutaneous coronary intervention). JACC Cardiovasc Interv. 2015;8:1704–14.
5. Ali ZA, Maehara A, Généreux P, Shlofmitz RA, Fabbiocchi F, Nazif TM, et al. Optical coherence tomography compared with intravascular ultrasound and with angiography to guide coronary stent implantation (ILUMIEN III: OPTIMIZE PCI): a randomised controlled trial. The Lancet. 2016;388 (10060):2618–28.
6. Prati F, Romagnoli E, Burzotta F, Limbruno U, Gatto L, La Manna A, et al. Clinical impact of OCT findings during PCI: the CLI-OPCI II study. JACC Cardiovasc Imaging. 2015;8:1297–305.
7. Romagnoli E, Sangiorgi GM, Cosgrave J, Guillet E, Colombo A. Drug-eluting stenting: the case for post-dilation. JACC Cardiovasc Interv. 2008;1:22–31.
8. Holmes DR Jr, Kereiakes DJ, Garg S, Serruys PW, Dehmer GJ, Ellis SG, et al. Stent thrombosis. J Am Coll Cardiol. 2010;56:1357–65.
9. van Werkum JW, Heestermans AA, de Korte FI, Kelder JC, Suttorp MJ, Rensing BJ, et al. Long-term clinical outcome after

a first angiographically confirmed coronary stent thrombosis: an analysis of 431 cases. Circulation. 2009;119:828–34.
10. Burzotta F, Parma A, Pristipino C, Manzoli A, Belloni F, Sardella G, et al. Angiographic and clinical outcome of invasively managed patients with thrombosed coronary bare metal or drug-eluting stents: the OPTIMIST study. Eur Heart J. 2008;29:3011–21.
11. Moreno R, Fernández C, Hernández R, Alfonso F, Angiolillo DJ, Sabaté M, et al. Drug-eluting stent thrombosis: results from a pooled analysis including 10 randomized studies. J Am Coll Cardiol. 2005;45:954–9.
12. Orford JL, Lennon R, Melby S, Fasseas P, Bell MR, Rihal CS, et al. Frequency and correlates of coronary stent thrombosis in the modern era: analysis of a single center registry. J Am Coll Cardiol. 2002;40:1567–72.
13. Iakovou I, Schmidt T, Bonizzoni E, Ge L, Sangiorgi GM, Stankovic G, et al. Incidence, predictors, and outcome of thrombosis after successful implantation of drug-eluting stents. JAMA. 2005;293:2126–30.
14. Fujii K, Carlier SG, Mintz GS, Yang YM, Moussa I, Weisz G, et al. Stent underexpansion and residual reference segment stenosis are related to stent thrombosis after sirolimus-eluting stent implantation: an intravascular ultrasound study. J Am Coll Cardiol. 2005;45:995–8.
15. Parodi G, La Manna A, Di Vito L, Valgimigli M, Fineschi M, Bellandi B, et al. Stent-related defects in patients presenting with stent thrombosis: differences at optical coherence tomography between subacute and late/very late thrombosis in the Mechanism Of Stent Thrombosis (MOST) study. EuroIntervention. 2013;9:936–44.
16. Cook S, Ladich E, Nakazawa G, Eshtehardi P, Neidhart M, Vogel R, et al. Correlation of intravascular ultrasound findings with histopathological analysis of thrombus aspirates in patients with very late drug-eluting stent thrombosis. Circulation. 2009;120:391–9.
17. Cook S, Wenaweser P, Togni M, Billinger M, Morger C, Seiler C, et al. Incomplete stent apposition and very late stent thrombosis after drug-eluting stent implantation. Circulation. 2007;115:2426–34.
18. Mega JL, Simon T, Collet JP, Anderson JL, Antman EM, Bliden K, et al. Reduced-function CYP2C19 genotype and risk of adverse clinical outcomes among patients treated with clopidogrel predominantly for PCI: a meta-analysis. JAMA. 2010;304:1821–30.
19. Airoldi F, Colombo A, Morici N, Latib A, Cosgrave J, Buellesfeld L, et al. Incidence and predictors of drug-eluting stent thrombosis during and after discontinuation of thienopyridine treatment. Circulation. 2007;116:745–54.
20. Alfonso F, Byrne RA, Rivero F, Kastrati A. Current treatment of in-stent restenosis. J Am Coll Cardiol. 2014;63:2659–73.
21. Kang SJ, Mintz GS, Park DW, Lee SW, Kim YH, Lee CW, et al. Tissue characterization of in-stent neointima using intravascular ultrasound radiofrequency data analysis. Am J Cardiol. 2010;106:1561–5.
22. Kang SJ, Mintz GS, Akasaka T, Park DW, Lee JY, Kim WJ, et al. Optical coherence tomographic analysis of in-stent neoatherosclerosis after drug-eluting stent implantation. Circulation. 2011;123:2954–63.
23. Lee SY, Hur SH, Lee SG, Kim SW, Shin DH, Kim JS, et al. Optical coherence tomographic observation of in-stent neoatherosclerosis in lesions with more than 50% neointimal area stenosis after second-generation drug-eluting stent implantation. Circ Cardiovasc Interv. 2015;8:e001878.
24. Nakazawa G, Otsuka F, Nakano M, Vorpahl M, Yazdani SK, Ladich E, et al. The pathology of neoatherosclerosis in human coronary implants bare-metal and drug-eluting stents. J Am Coll Cardiol. 2011;57:1314–22.
25. Alfonso F, Sandoval J, Nolte C. Calcified in-stent restenosis: a rare cause of dilation failure requiring rotational atherectomy. Circ Cardiovasc Interv. 2012;5:e1–2.
26. Bastante T, Rivero F, Cuesta J, Alfonso F. Calcified neoatherosclerosis causing "undilatable" in-stent restenosis: insights of optical coherence tomography and role of rotational atherectomy. JACC Cardiovasc Interv. 2015;8:2039–40.
27. Ali ZA, Roleder T, Narula J, Mohanty BD, Baber U, Kovacic JC, et al. Increased thin-cap neoatheroma and periprocedural myocardial infarction in drug-eluting stent restenosis: multimodality intravascular imaging of drug-eluting and bare-metal stents. Circ Cardiovasc Interv. 2013;6:507–17.

5 New Stents, New Procedures, and Intraprocedural Challenges

5.1 Introduction

The current generation of drug eluting stents (DESs) has several advantages over the previous generations of DESs and bare metal stents (BMSs) and offers good efficacy and safety. However, the risk of stent thrombosis remains, and the stented vessel remains permanently associated with a rigid metal cage. Bioresorbable vascular scaffolds (BRSs) have recently reenergized the field of coronary intervention; they support transient drug delivery and vessel patency and then gradually tend to complete resorption [1, 2]. Therefore, BRSs might allow restoration of vasomotion and distensibility [3] and may exclude stent thrombosis, "jailing" of the side branches, and struts overhanging over ostial lesions. They may also obviate the inability to surgically graft stented segments [4]. Optical coherence tomography (OCT) has played a major role in the development of BRS technology by providing more precise and detailed morphologic information (compared to IVUS) as a result of its higher resolution [5–8]. While the clinical outcome data from the landmark BRS trials are promising [9–11], the studies had numerous limitations regarding patient and lesion selection. There are a paucity of data on BRS implantation in unselected patient population in "real world" clinical practice, including in-stent restenosis, bifurcation, and severely calcified lesions [12–14]. Similar to metallic stents, suboptimal implantation with incomplete lesion coverage, scaffold underexpansion, and strut malapposition have been the main pathomechanisms for both early and late BRS thrombosis [15]. OCT imaging can help optimize BRS sizing and guide postdilation in order to avoid scaffold underexpansion or fracture.

For metallic stents, OCT has demonstrated exquisite capability to clarify abnormal angiographic findings, including peristrut contrast staining and intraluminal filling defects. Abnormal coronary dilatation at the site of DES implantation demonstrating contrast staining outside the stent struts, peri-stent contrast staining (PSS), has been shown to be associated with target-lesion revascularization and very late stent thrombosis [16]. OCT can differentiate between two main underlying causes of PSS, incomplete stent apposition and multiple interstrut hollows or cavities between well apposed stent struts [17]. Intraluminal filling defects are occasionally observed on coronary angiography, and thrombosis has often been used as a default diagnosis; however, there are many different causes responsible for the phenomenon, including calcification, dissection, plaque rupture, and artifacts [18]. OCT allows accurate characterization angiographic filling defects and provides important information for treatment optimization.

Electronic Supplementary Material The online version of this chapter (doi:10.1007/978-3-319-62666-6_5) contains supplementary material, which is available to authorized users.

A. Kini et al., *Atlas of Coronary Intravascular Optical Coherence Tomography*, DOI 10.1007/978-3-319-62666-6_5

5.2 Case 1. Preparing a Heavily Calcified Lesion for Accepting a Bioresorbable Vascular Scaffold (Figs. 5.1 and 5.2, Videos 5.1 and 5.2)

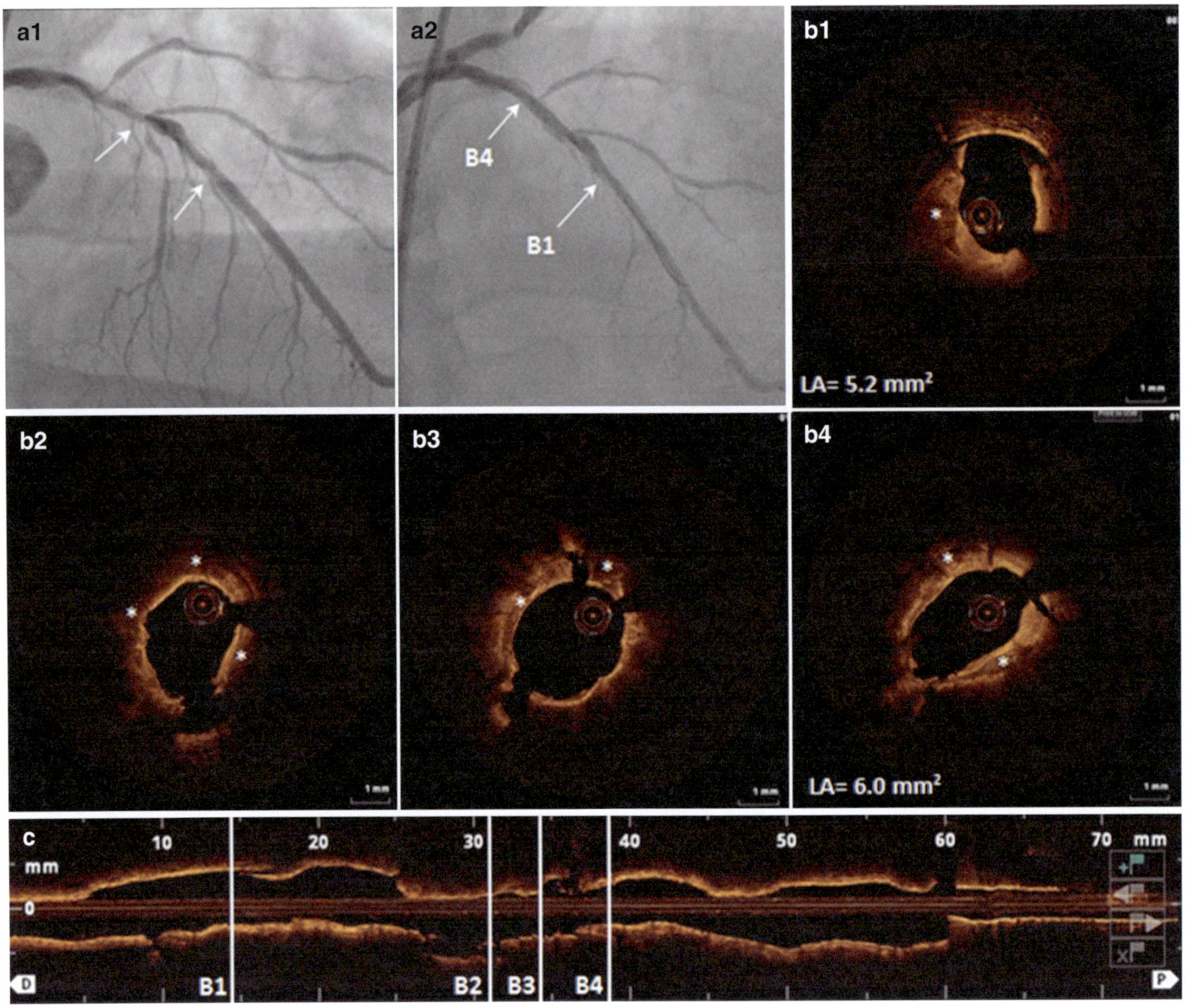

Fig. 5.1 A 78-year-old male, an ex-smoker with hyperlipidemia, controlled hypertension, and positive stress cardiovascular magnetic resonance imaging (CMR) presented with stable angina. Coronary angiography showed severely calcified stenoses in the proximal and mid LAD (**a1**, *arrows*). To ablate calcified plaque, rotational atherectomy (RA) was performed with a 1.75-mm burr at 160,000 rpm for 88 s resulting in significant lumen gain by angiography (**a2**). OCT pullback after atherectomy verified effective calcium debulking by visualizing significant modifications of fibrocalcific plaques (**b1**–**b4**, *asterisks*) with minimal lumen area (LA) of 6.0 (**b4**) and 5.2 mm^2 (**b1**) in the proximal and distal segments respectively

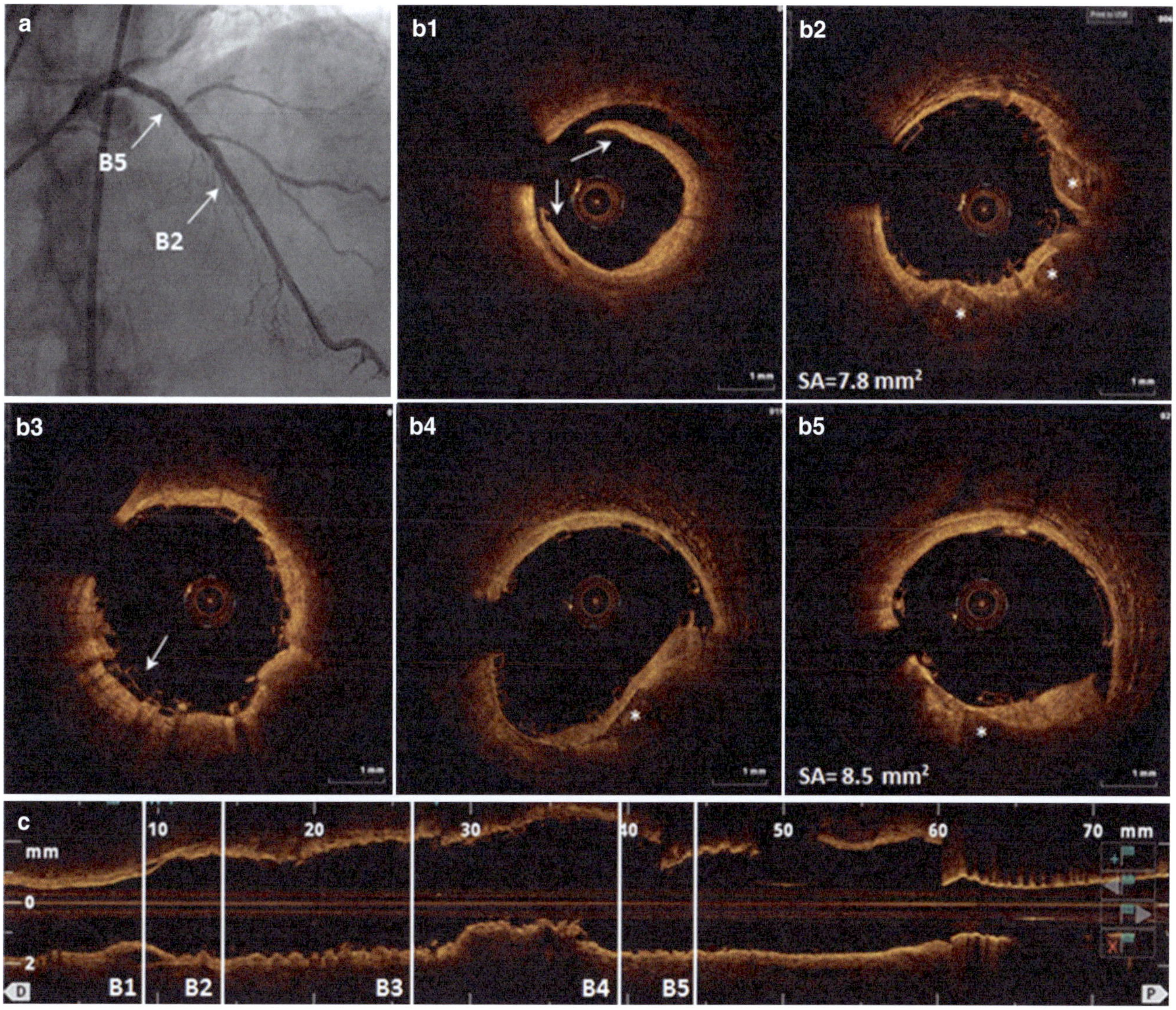

Fig. 5.2 Coronary angiography and OCT imaging after BRS implantation. Two BRS, 3.5/28- and 3.5/18-mm, were deployed in the proximal and mid LAD with a satisfactory angiographic result (**a**). OCT pullback confirmed good scaffold expansion and apposition (**b2**, **b4**, **b5**) with the minimal scaffold area (SA) of 7.8 and 8.5 mm² and a short (1.6 mm) scaffold overlap segment (**b3**, *arrow*). At the distal edge of the distal BRS, OCT detected a 2.4-mm intima-media dissection (**b1**, *arrows*), which was successfully treated with an additional 3.25/12-mm DES. In this case, OCT helped assess the effectiveness of calcium ablation and an immediate post-PCI complication not detected by angiography

5.3 Case 2. Preparing a Totally Occluded Vessel for a Bioresorbable Vascular Scaffold (Figs. 5.3 and 5.4, Videos 5.3 and 5.4)

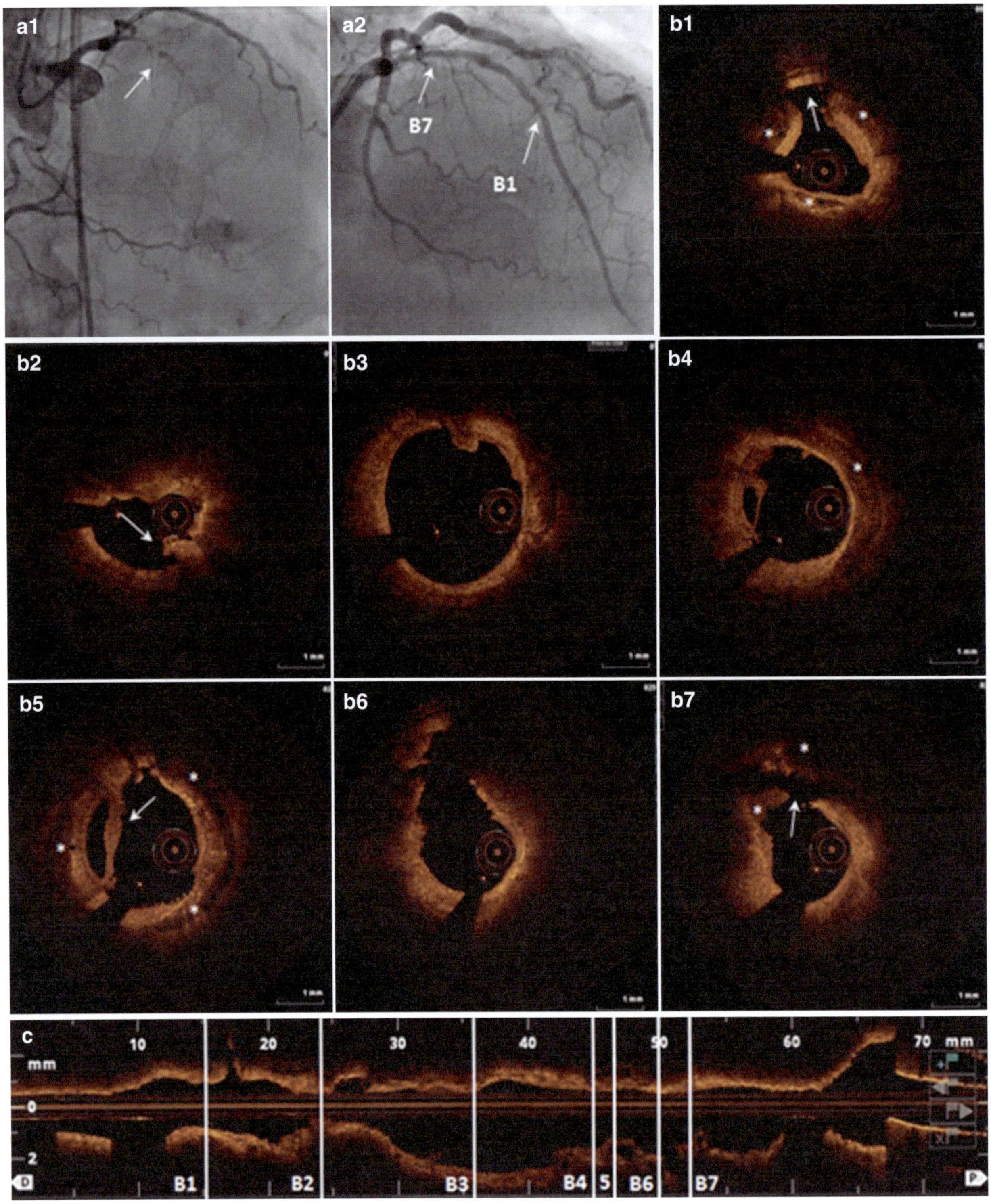

Fig. 5.3 A 67-year-old male with controlled hyperlipidemia, hypertension, and NIDDM presented with worsening chest pain. Single photon emission computed tomography myocardial perfusion imaging (SPECT-MPI) demonstrated moderate ischemia in the mid LAD area. Coronary angiography showed severely calcified proximal LAD chronic total occlusion (CTO) with collateral flow from the RCA (**a1**, *arrow*). CTO was successfully crossed using the antegrade approach with a Fielder wire. Orbital atherectomy was performed in the proximal and mid LAD with 1.25-mm burr at 80,000 rpm for 60 s. OCT pullback performed after lesion predilatation by a noncompliant balloon revealed almost circumferential calcification in the proximal (**b4**–**b7**, *asterisks*) and middle (**b1**, *asterisks*) portions of the LAD and visualized significant modifications of fibrocalcific plaques (*arrows*)

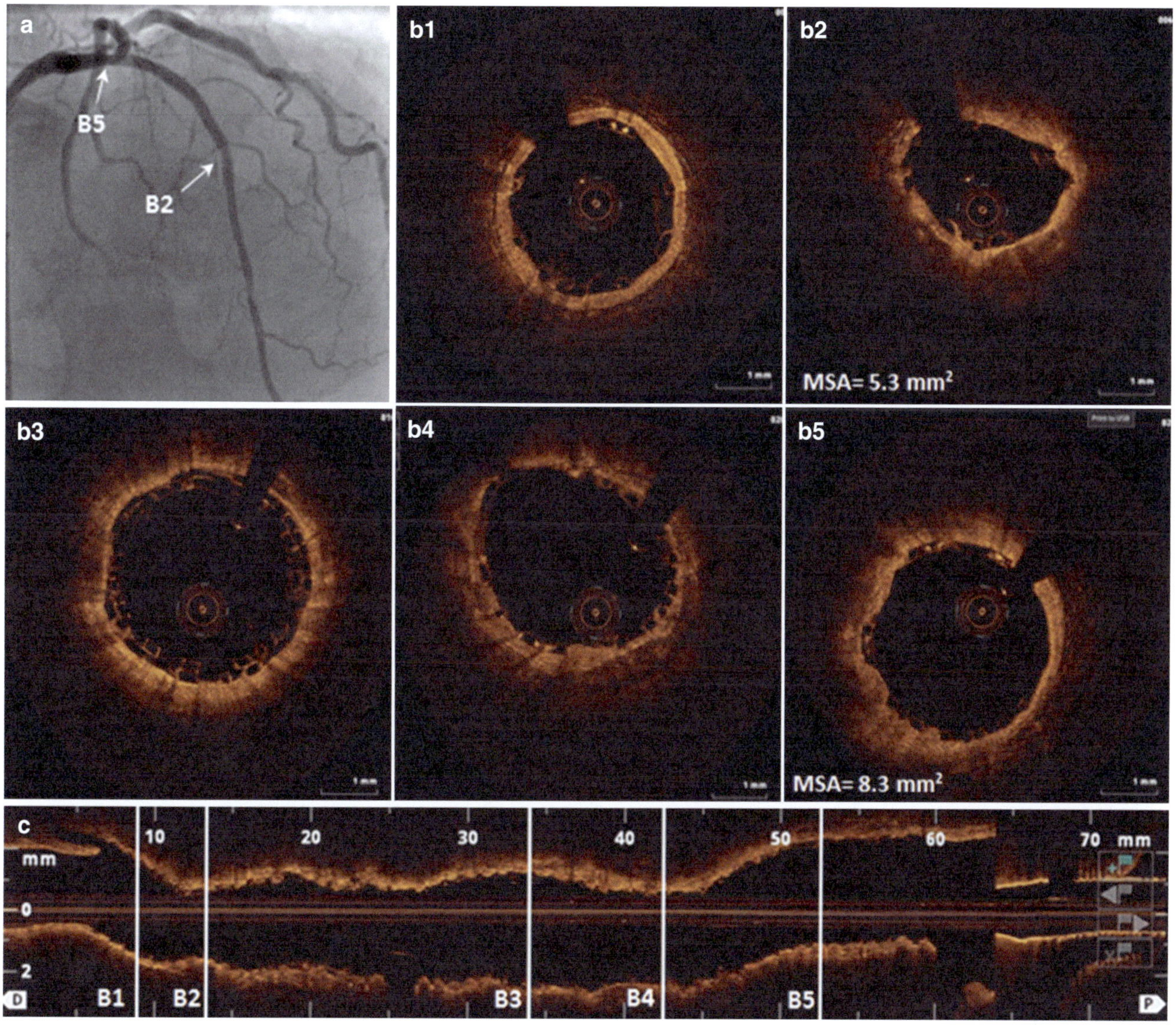

Fig. 5.4 Post-stent imaging. To cover the entire diseased segment, two BRSs were implanted in the proximal (3.5/28 mm) and mid (3.0/28 mm) LAD followed by postdilation with a 3.5-mm noncompliant balloon at 20 atm with satisfactory result by angiography (**a**). Postprocedural OCT showed good expansion and apposition for both scaffolds without any evidence for dissection or strut malapposition in the whole stented segment with a 1.6-mm long overlap segment (**b3**). The minimal area of the proximal and distal scaffold was 8.3 and 5.3 mm^2 respectively. In the present case, OCT demonstrated BRS implantation in a calcified CTO lesion with good results for scaffold expansion and apposition after adequate lesion preparation and postdilatation

5.4 Case 3. Explaining the Unexplainable (Fig. 5.5, Video 5.5)

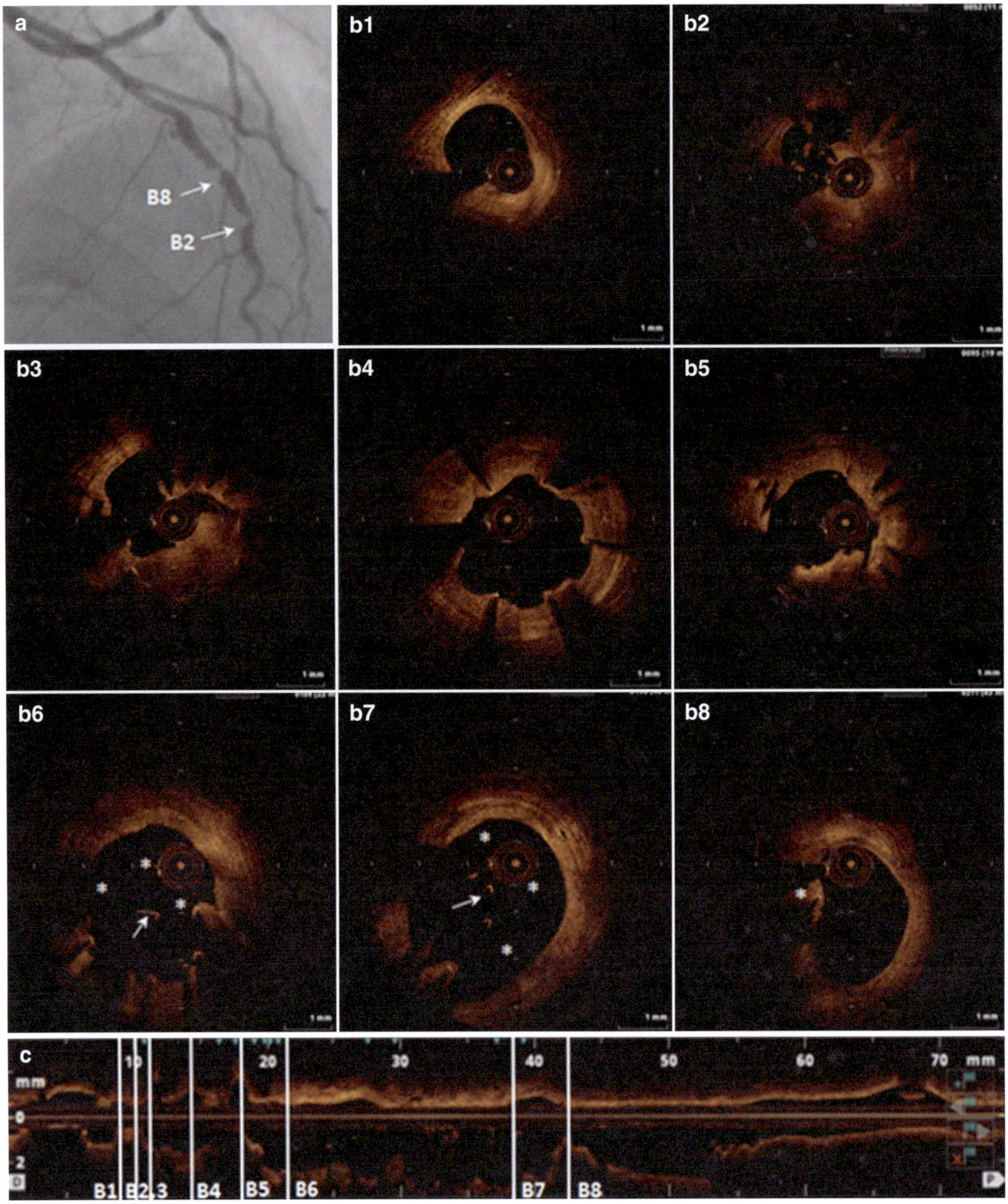

Fig. 5.5 A 52-year-old female ex-smoker with a history of multiple PCI and MI presented with CCS Class II angina and throat tightness after walking. Coronary computed tomography angiography (CCTA) suggested a possible in-stent restenosis of two DES stents (2.5/33 and 2.5/8 mm) implanted in the LAD in the setting of an MI 6 years earlier. Coronary angiography showed in-stent restenosis lesions in the mid LAD with peri-stent contrast staining suggesting a possibility of stent fracture (**a**). OCT pullback revealed proximal stent malapposition with a large distance between stent struts and the vessel wall (**b6**, **b7**, *asterisks*). The longitudinal length of the segment with incomplete strut apposition was 16 mm. The proximal edge of the stent was totally occluded (**b8**, *asterisk*), which prevented the guidewire from going inside the stent (**b6**, **b7**). The guidewire was observed inside the second distal stent, suggesting that there was either a gap between the two stents or a stent fracture at the site of the overlap. The distal stent shown in frames **b2** to **b5** appeared to be well expanded, but there was a focal in-stent restenosis lesion with an almost occluded distal edge (**b2**). Multiple interstrut cavities between well apposed stent struts were observed in the segment (**b4**). The imaging catheter was located inside the distal stent. Further treatment including surgical option for revascularization was discussed with the Heart Team, and robotic CABG with LIMA to LAD was performed 2 weeks after the visit. In this case, OCT helped characterize the etiology of PSS on angiography and provided detailed information on morphology of the lesion for the Heart Team

5.5 Case 4. Clarifying the Halos (Figs. 5.6 and 5.7, Videos 5.6 and 5.7)

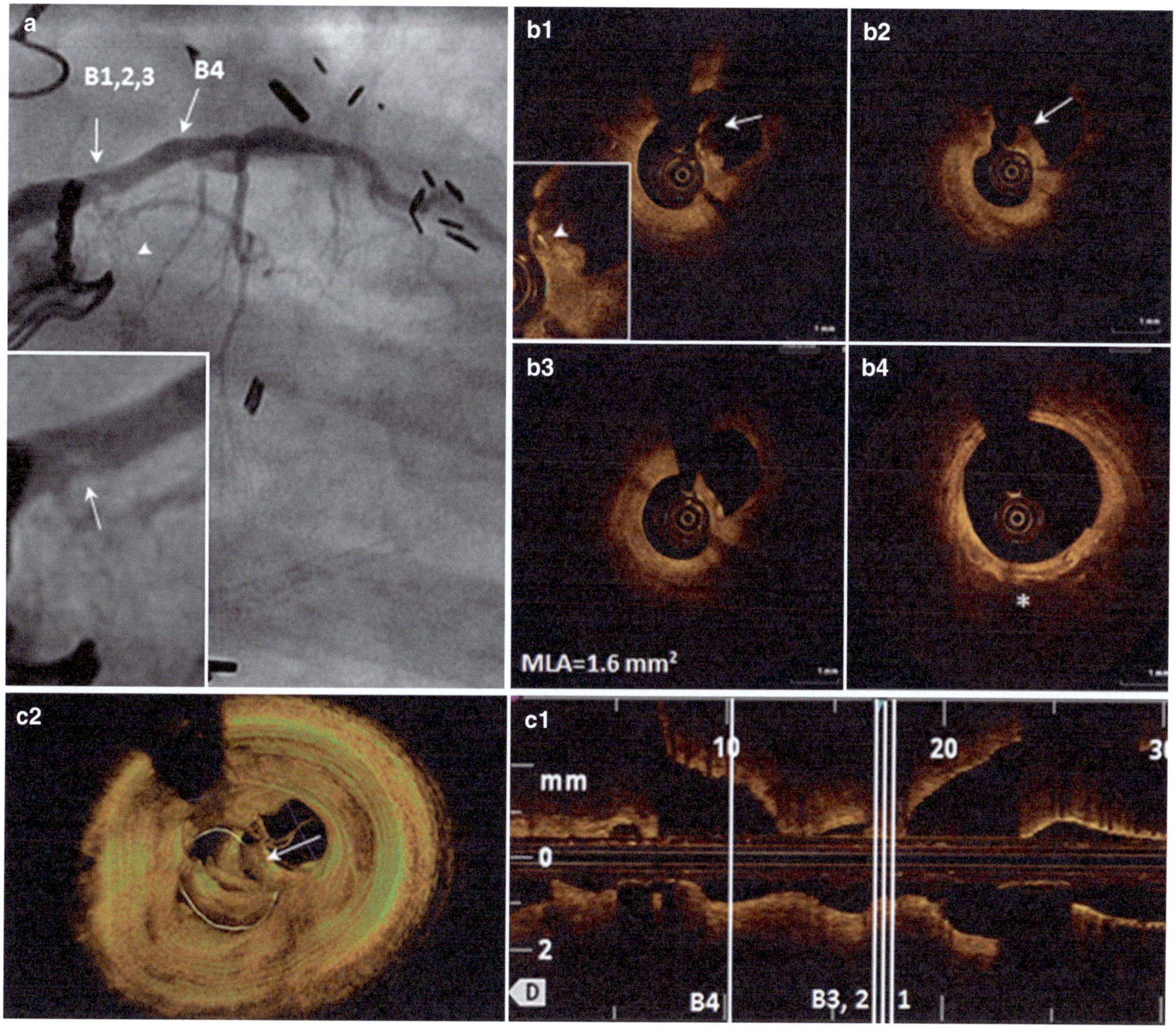

Fig. 5.6 A 52-year-old female with controlled hypertension, IDDM, hyperlipidemia, and a prior history of multiple PCI, CABG, and abnormal SPECT-MPI presented to the Emergency Department with chest pain and shortness of breath on exertion. The last PCI was performed 4 years earlier with an evelolimus eluting stent implanted in the proximal LCX. Computed tomography (CT) of the chest showed patent LIMA and an occluded LCX stent. Coronary angiography showed an intermediate stenosis with an intraluminal filling defect in the ostial LAD (**a**-*inset, arrow*) and confirmed total occlusion of LCX filling with collaterals from RCA and LAD (**a**, *arrowhead*). OCT pullback of the LAD detected a healed plaque rupture in the ostial LAD (**b1**, **b2**, *arrows*), significant stenosis with an MLA of 1.6 mm^2 (**b3**), and a two-quadrant calcification distal to MLA (**b4**, *asterisk*). One strut of the LCX stent can be visualized in OCT frame **b1** (*inset, arrowhead*), suggesting that the plaque might be a part of the ISR lesion in the proximal LCX. Three-dimensional OCT reconstruction (**c2**) allows better visualization of the ruptured plaque cavity (*circled*) and ruptured fibrous cap (*arrow*). Since there was no thrombotic mass detected in the lesion, dye trapped within the cavity is the most probable cause of the filling defect. Based on the OCT detection of significant stenosis, the lesion was treated with a new stent implantation

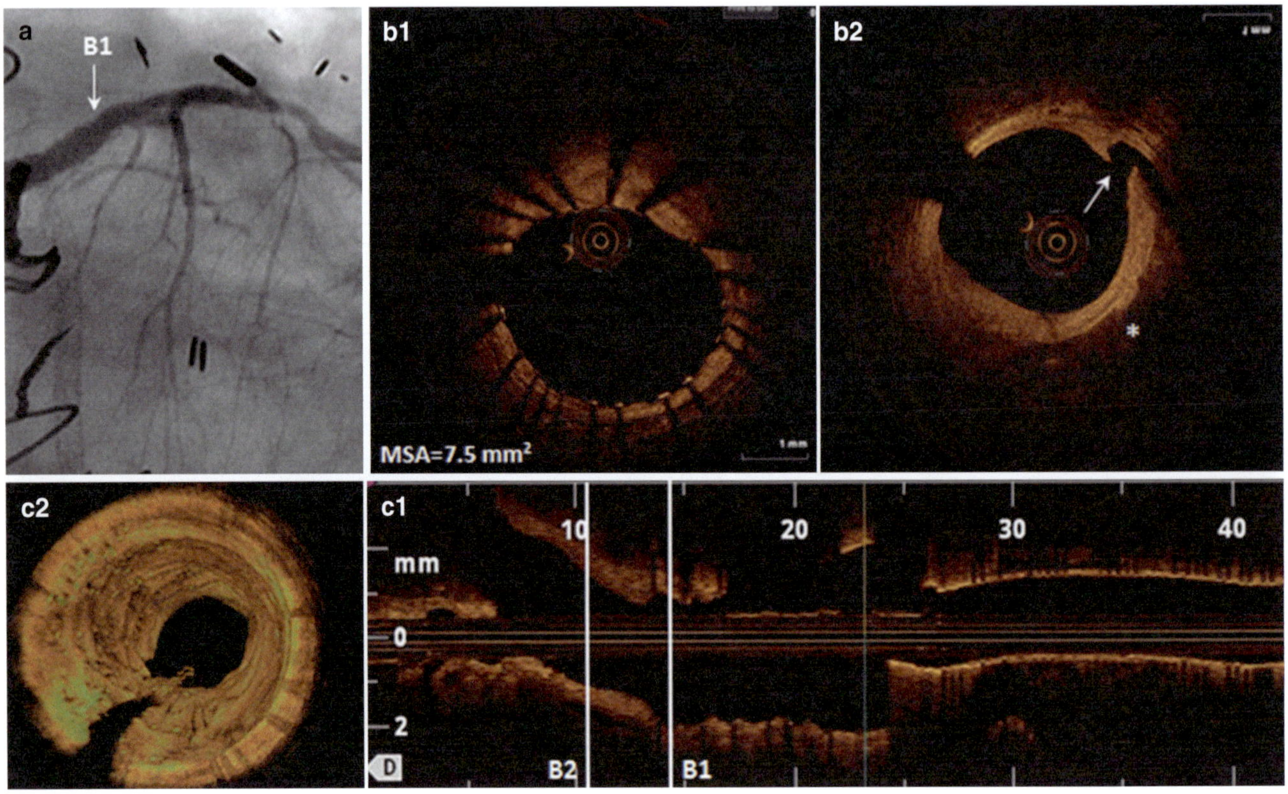

Fig. 5.7 Final poststent angiogram and OCT pullback. A 4/12-mm everolimus eluting stent was deployed into the LAD with good angiographic result (**a**), verified by two-dimensional (**b1**) and three-dimensional (**c2**) OCT. A distal stent edge dissection (**b2**, *arrow*) visualized by OCT around calcified plaque (**b2**, *asterisk*) was left untreated. In this case, OCT detected healed plaque rupture as the underlying cause of the angiographic filling defect, which led to an additional stent implantation

5.6 Case 5. I Cannot Possibly Muddy the Water You Are Drinking Up There (Figs. 5.8, 5.9 and 5.10, Videos 5.8, 5.9 and 5.10)

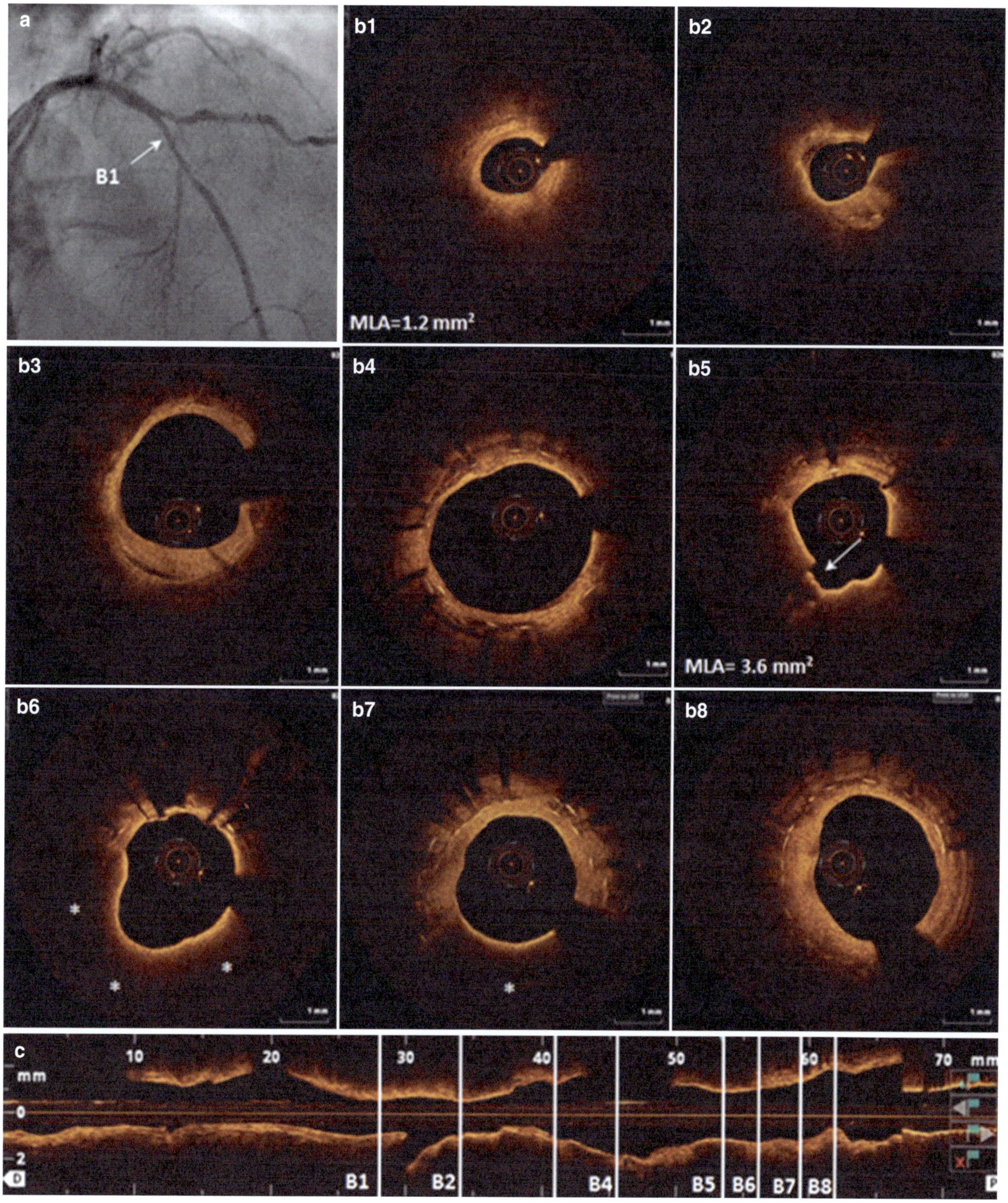

Fig. 5.8 A 52-year-old male who was an ex-smoker with controlled IDDM, hyperlipidemia, and a history of multiple PCI presented for a staged intervention of the mid LAD. Angiography showed a patent stent in the proximal LAD and a 60–70% stenosis in the mid portion of the vessel (**a**). OCT images of the LAD demonstrated a large lipid plaque with extensive macrophage accumulation around the bifurcation area (**b1**, **b2**) and mostly fibrocalcific plaque proximal to the MLA (**b3**). The same OCT pullback allowed visualization of two stents previously implanted in the proximal LAD (**b4**–**b8**). A lipid-rich plaque with a thin fibrous cap was detected inside the stents (**b5**–**b7**, *asterisks*) with a possible fibrous cap rupture site detected at the proximal LAD minimal lumen area frame (**b5**, *arrow*). Mostly fibrocalcific neointima was visualized in the distal and proximal edges of the proximal LAD stent

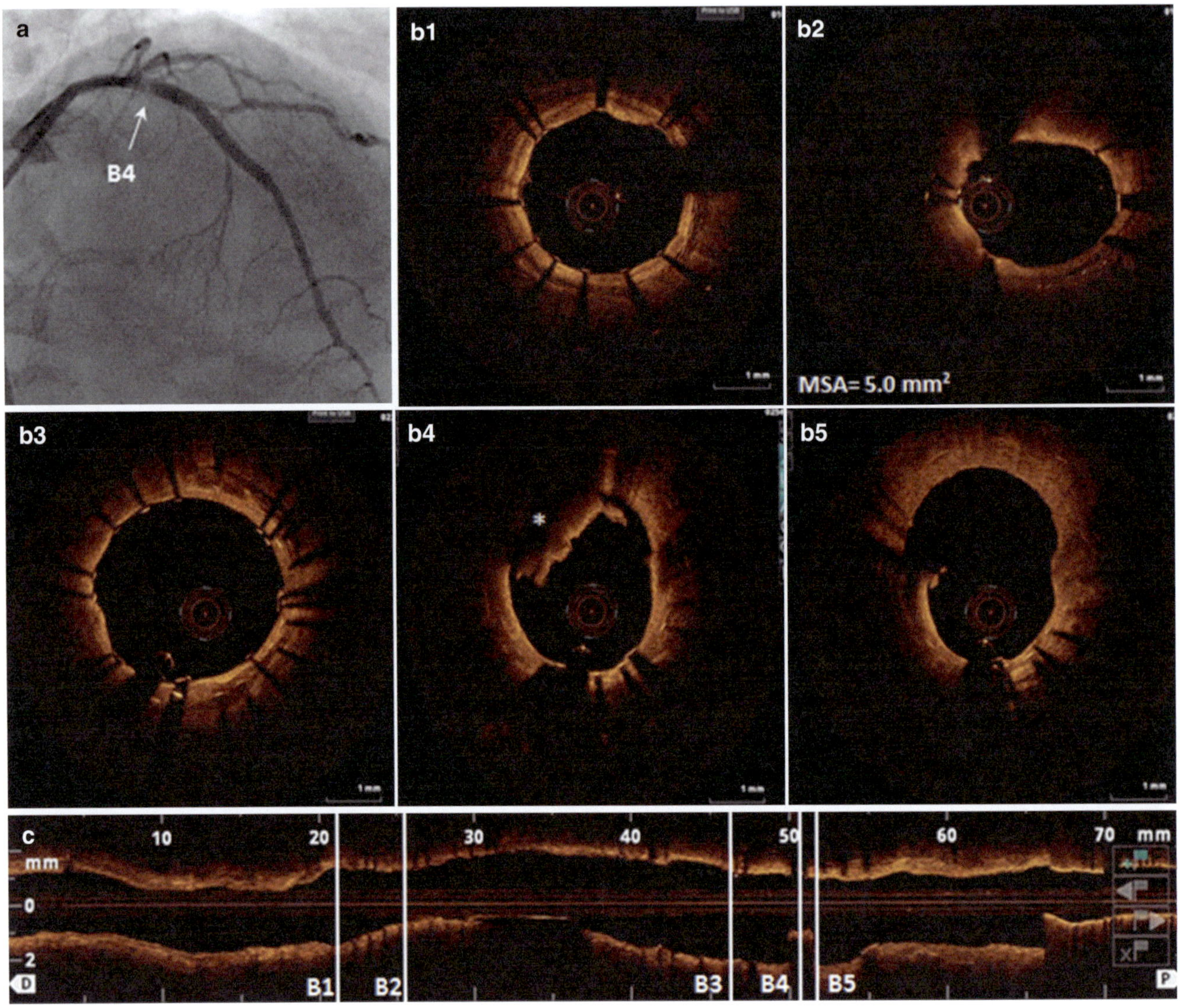

Fig. 5.9 Coronary angiography and OCT after mid LAD stenting. After a 3.5/28-mm everolimus-eluting stent was implanted in the mid LAD, an intraluminal filling defect was noted on the angiogram (**a**, *arrow*). OCT detected new thrombus formation within the proximal stent (**b4**, *asterisk*) probably caused by plaque rupture. Based on the OCT findings, a decision was made to perform PTCA of the proximal segment using 3.75/12-mm noncompliant balloon

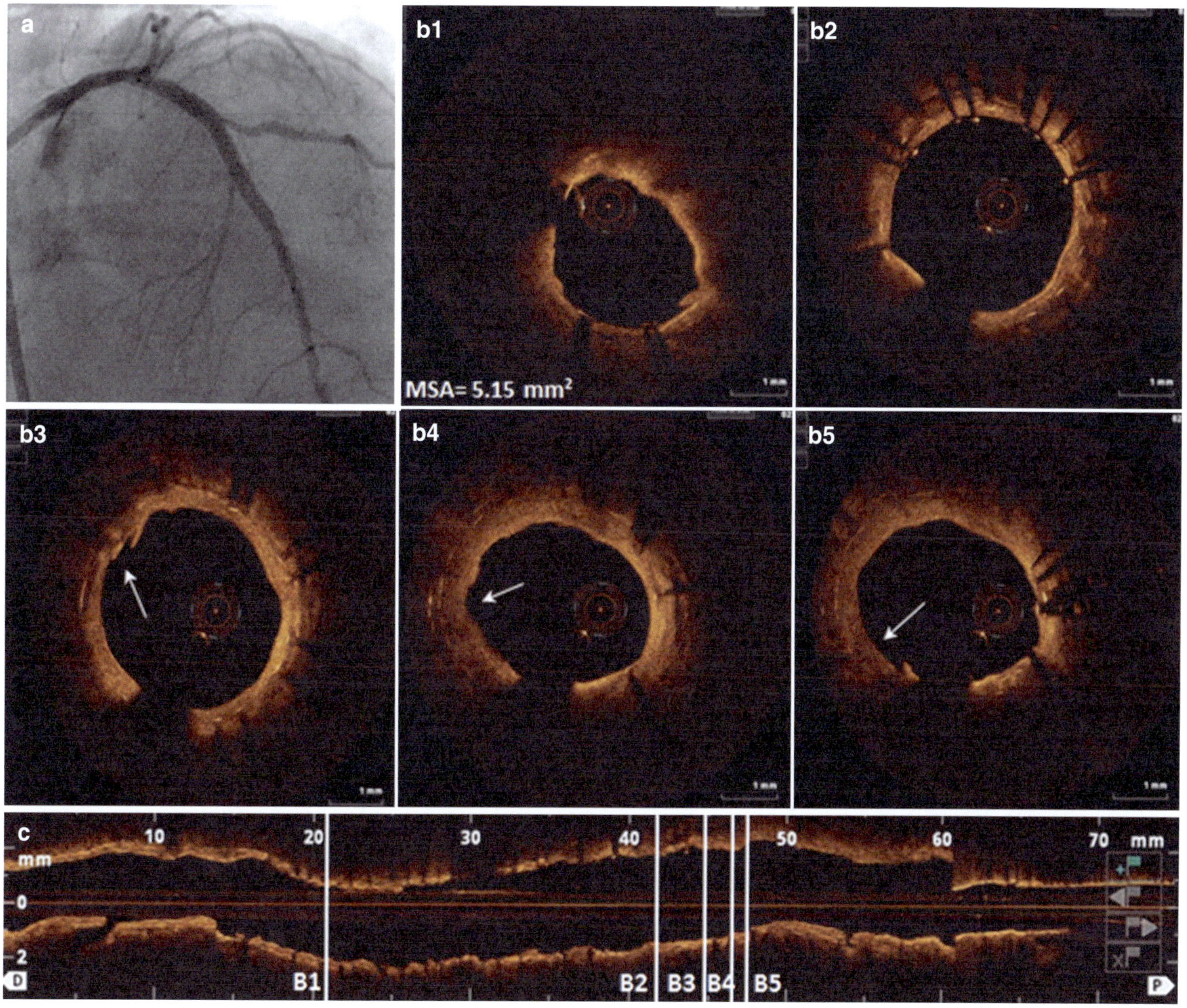

Fig. 5.10 Final post-PCI imaging. While there was no remaining thrombotic mass detected after postdilatation, OCT visualized lumen surface irregularities at the site of the thrombus formation (**b3**–**b5**, *arrows*). In this case, OCT helped clarify the etiology of the angiographic intraluminal filling defect and to select a noncompliant balloon PTCA as the treatment strategy

References

1. Serruys PW, Garcia-Garcia HM, Onuma Y. From metallic cages to transient bioresorbable scaffolds: change in paradigm of coronary revascularization in the upcoming decade? Eur Heart J. 2012;33:16–25b.
2. Waksman R. Biodegradable stents: they do their job and disappear. J Invasive Cardiol. 2006;18:70–4.
3. Brugaletta S, Heo JH, Garcia-Garcia HM, Farooq V, van Geuns RJ, de Bruyne B, et al. Endothelial-dependent vasomotion in a coronary segment treated by ABSORB everolimus-eluting bioresorbable vascular scaffold system is related to plaque composition at the time of bioresorption of the polymer: indirect finding of vascular reparative therapy? Eur Heart J. 2012;33:1325–33.
4. Okamura T, Serruys PW, Regar E. Cardiovascular flashlight. The fate of bioresorbable struts located at a side branch ostium: serial three-dimensional optical coherence tomography assessment. Eur Heart J. 2010;31:2179.
5. Gomez-Lara J, Brugaletta S, Farooq V, Onuma Y, Diletti R, Windecker S, et al. Head-to-head comparison of the neointimal response between metallic and bioresorbable everolimus-eluting scaffolds using optical coherence tomography. JACC Cardiovasc Interv. 2011;4:1271–80.
6. Karanasos A, Simsek C, Gnanadesigan M, Nienke S, van Ditzhuijzen MSC, et al. OCT assessment of the long-term vascular healing response 5 years after everolimus-eluting bioresorbable vascular scaffold. J Am Coll Cardiol. 2014;64:2343–56.
7. Mattesini A, Secco GG, Dall'Ara G, Ghione M, Rama-Merchan JC, Lupi A, et al. ABSORB biodegradable stents versus second-generation metal stents: a comparison study of 100 complex lesions treated under OCT guidance. JACC Cardiovasc Interv. 2014;7:741–50.
8. Zhang YJ, Iqbal J, Nakatani S, Bourantas CV, Campos C, Ishibashi Y, et al. Scaffold and edge vascular response following implantation of everolimus-eluting bioresorbable vascular scaffold: a 3-year serial optical coherence tomography study. JACC Cardiovasc Interv. 2014;7:1361–9.
9. Serruys PW, Onuma Y, Dudek D, Smits PC, Koolen J, Chevalier B, et al. Evaluation of the second generation of a bioresorbable everolimus-eluting vascular scaffold for the treatment of de novo coronary artery stenosis: 12-month clinical and imaging outcomes. J Am Coll Cardiol. 2011;58:1578–88.
10. Diletti R, Serruys PW, Farooq V, Sudhir K, Dorange C, Miquel-Sudhir K, et al. ABSORB II randomized controlled trial: a clinical evaluation to compare the safety, efficacy, and performance of the Absorb everolimus-eluting bioresorbable vascular scaffold system against the XIENCE everolimus-eluting coronary stent system in the treatment of subjects with ischemic heart disease caused by de novo native coronary artery lesions: rationale and study design. Am Heart J. 2012;164:654–63.
11. Ellis SG, Kereiakes DJ, Metzger DC, Caputo RP, Rizik DG, Teirstein PS, et al. Everolimus-eluting bioresorbable scaffolds for coronary artery disease. N Engl J Med. 2015;373:1905–15.
12. Capodanno D, Gori T, Nef H, Latib A, Mehilli J, Lesiak M, et al. Percutaneous coronary intervention with everolimus-eluting bioresorbable vascular scaffolds in routine clinical practice: early and midterm outcomes from the European multicentre GHOST-EU registry. EuroIntervention. 2015;10:1144–53.
13. Kawamoto H, Ruparelia N, Figini F, Latib A, Colombo A. Severe neointimal hyperplasia of neoplastic carina following bioresorbable scaffold implantation using t-stenting and small protrusion technique: insights from optical frequency domain imaging. JACC Cardiovasc Interv. 2015;8:e207–9.
14. Capranzano P, Francaviglia B, Capodanno D, Di Salvo ME, Tamburino CI, Santagati FM, et al. Embolization of fractured bioresorbable scaffold struts: insights from 2- and 3-dimensional optical coherence tomography. JACC Cardiovasc Interv. 2016; 9:e37–8.
15. Karanasos A, Van Mieghem N, van Ditzhuijzen N, Felix C, Daemen J, Autar A, et al. Angiographic and optical coherence tomography insights into bioresorbable scaffold thrombosis: single-center experience. Circ Cardiovasc Interv. 2015;8(5). pii: e002369. doi: 10.1161/CIRCINTERVENTIONS.114.002369.
16. Imai M, Kadota K, Goto T, Fujii S, Yamamoto H, Fuku Y, et al. Incidence, risk factors, and clinical sequelae of angiographic peri-stent contrast staining after sirolimus-eluting stent implantation. Circulation. 2011;123:2382–91.
17. Tada T, Kadota K, Hosogi S, Kubo S, Ozaki M, Yoshino M, et al. Optical coherence tomography findings in lesions after sirolimus-eluting stent implantation with peri-stent contrast staining. Circ Cardiovasc Interv. 2012;5:649–56.
18. Jaffe R, Irfan A, Hong T, Chisholm RJ, Cheema AN. Intraluminal filling defects on coronary angiography: more than meets the eye. Clin Cardiol. 2007;30:480–4.

Index

A. Kini et al., *Atlas of Coronary Intravascular Optical Coherence Tomography*, DOI 10.1007/978-3-319-62666-6

MIX
Papier aus verantwortungsvollen Quellen
Paper from responsible sources
FSC® C105338

If you have any concerns about our products,
you can contact us on
ProductSafety@springernature.com

In case Publisher is established outside the EU,
the EU authorized representative is:
Springer Nature Customer Service Center GmbH
Europaplatz 3, 69115 Heidelberg, Germany

Printed by Libri Plureos GmbH
in Hamburg, Germany